# State of Vaccination

## New Perspectives in South Asian History 24

The **New Perspectives in South Asian History** series publishes monographs and other writings on early modern, modern and contemporary history. The volumes in the series cover new ground across a broad spectrum of subjects such as cultural, environmental, medical, military and political history, and the histories of 'marginalised' groups. It includes fresh perspectives on more familiar fields as well as interdisciplinary and original work from all parts of South Asia. It welcomes historical contributions from sociology, anthropology and cultural studies.

# *State of Vaccination*

## *The Fight Against Smallpox in Colonial Burma*

Atsuko Naono
*University of Warwick*

Orient BlackSwan

The Wellcome Trust Centre for the History of Medicine at University College London
www.ucl.ac.uk/histmed · 020 7679 8100
UCL

**ORIENT BLACKSWAN PRIVATE LIMITED**

*Registered Office*
3-6-752 Himayatnagar, Hyderabad 500 029 (A.P.), India
E-mail: centraloffice@orientblackswan.com

*Other Offices*
Bangalore, Bhopal, Bhubaneshwar, Chennai,
Ernakulam, Guwahati, Hyderabad, Jaipur, Kolkata,
Lucknow, Mumbai, New Delhi, Patna


First Published 2009



ISBN 978 81 250 3546 6

*Typeset by*
OSDATA, Hyderabad 500 029
in Bembo (Aldine) 10.5/12.5

*Printed at*
Graphica Printers
Hyderabad 500 013

*Published by*
Orient Blackswan Private Limited
3-6-752 Himayatnagar, Hyderabad 500 029 (A.P.), India
Email: hyderabad@orientblackswan.com

The publishers gratefully acknowledge the financial support received for this volume from the Wellcome Trust Centre for the History of Medicine at University College London.

*To My Parents*

# *Contents*

# *List of Maps*

# *List of Tables*

# *List of Appendices*

# Acknowledgements

My initial understanding of Burma was developed under the careful guidance of Ryuji Okudaira and Teruko Saito during my undergraduate days (and after) at the Tokyo University of Foreign Studies. I became interested in smallpox vaccination in colonial Burma while doing my doctoral studies at the University of Michigan under Victor B. Lieberman (Vic) and Rudolf Mrazek (Rudy). Rudy stimulated my interest in the colonial period, especially for the colonial mode of things that could not be separated from human agency. Vic, aside from strengthening my understanding of Burmese history, showed me the importance of the role of administrative structures and encouraged me to look broadly at developments across regions rather than only within Burma. Over the course of my study at Michigan, I was fortunate to have the opportunity of being instructed and guided by other scholars, including Leslie Pincus, Joel D. Howell, Martin S. Pernick, Hitomi Tonomura, John K. Whitmore, and Nancy K. Florida, who in one way or another contributed to either my understanding of Southeast Asian history or the history of science, medicine, and technology, or both. I had studied Burmese during my undergraduate years in Tokyo but I further developed my abilities in the Burmese language through summer studies at the University of Wisconsin-Madison under U Saw Tun, San San Hnin Tun, John Okell, and Than Than Win.

I have been very fortunate to have met many other people over the years who gave me valuable suggestions, advice, help, time, and encouragement, and directed me to useful sources. Special thanks is owed to Daw Sandar Win, U Thaw Kaung, U Naing Aung, Keiko Tosa, Peter Boomgaard, Andrew Goss, Pax Bobrow, the late Daw May Kyi Win, Geoff Wade, Will Womack, Yuri Takahashi, Akio Takahashi, Natsuko Hayashi, Takizawa Toshiyuki, Hong Liu, Jon Fernquest, Monique Skidmore, Mya Mo Thu, and many others. Also, I am very grateful to Sanjoy Bhattacharya and Mark Harrison for encouraging me to publish my dissertation on which this book is based. My gratitude also goes to Veenu Luthria and Anil Menon at Orient Blackswan for help in easing the transition from manuscript to book and the anonymous referee(s) for their important suggestions in revising the manuscript. Sanjoy also read some of the chapters and provided invaluable comments. Hal Cook and Justin Watkins helped me in linking up with the Wellcome Centre for the History of Medicine at University College London and the Centre for Southeast Asian Studies at the School of Oriental and African Studies (SOAS), where I was able to continue my research and attend workshops and seminars from which I benefited greatly.

My appreciation also goes to many others for help along the way. These include many Burmese friends whose generosity and willingness to help always overwhelmed me. In Burma, I was always amazed at how quickly one was directed and introduced to others who could provide just the right kind of help. The help of staff at the following libraries and archives should also be mentioned: the Asia and African Studies Collection (formerly the Oriental and India Office Collection) at the British Library, the British Library's newspaper collection at Colindale, the Wellcome Library, the SOAS Library, the Central Library at Yangon University, the National Archives of Myanmar, the National University of Singapore Library, the Institute of Southeast Asian Studies Library, the Medical School Library at the University of Tokyo, the Toyo Bunko, the National Diet Library in Tokyo, and the Rackham Graduate and Public Health libraries at the University of Michigan. Last, I owe my greatest debt to my life partner, Mike Charney, for his patience and support, and to my parents and grandparents in Japan. I do not know how many sleepless nights I put them through.

## *List of Abbreviations*

| | |
|---|---|
| IMS | Indian Medical Service |
| MAMS | Myanmar Academy of Medical Science |
| NAUM | National Archives of the Union of Myanmar (Yangon) |
| OIOC | Oriental and India Office Collection. British Library (London) |

# Introduction

One of the difficulties of writing about the medical establishment in British India is the diversity of "India's ethnic, epidemiological, and administrative" make-up, as one scholar on the history of public health in the subcontinent put it.[1] Even when attempts to make thematic sense of this diversity are made, it is mainly data from the major provinces, especially the presidencies, and their contexts that inform the broad treatments that result. Compared to many other areas that were a part of British India, Burma is usually forgotten and rarely figures in studies of colonial health in the British Empire, which until 1937 (when Burma was separated from British India) stretched from Aden in the southern Arabian peninsula to the northern reaches of the Straits of Melaka. Burma presents a useful countervailing example of medicine under the Raj, one that highlights incongruities between the colonial medicine practised on the subcontinent and on its periphery.

Indigenous health in Burma was never a high priority for the British colonial government. Strategic and economic concerns motivated the region's incorporation into British India over the course of three wars in the nineteenth century. Burma was seen partly as a buffer against French Indochina and partly as a potential direct route to China's large market. Further, its rich natural resources, in particular timber and oil, and the rice produced in the delta area, prompted the British colonial government to organise the colonial state on lines that suited its commercial exploitation. Mary Callahan, in her study of the rise of the military as an institution from the colonial period to the early years of independence, revisits John Sydenham Furnivall's observation that colonial society in Burma was organised "for production", and points out that its

[1] Mark Harrison, *Public Health in British India: Anglo-Indian Preventive Medicine, 1859–1914* (Cambridge: Cambridge University Press, 1994), 1.

reordering to facilitate production and commerce proceeded with unprecedented speed, blindly transplanting administrative models developed on the subcontinent into Burma.[2] This was also true of the colonial medical establishment in Burma, which borrowed its organisation, methods, outlook, and even its personnel, from the other side of the Bay of Bengal.

Early colonial vaccination policies in Burma were thus strongly influenced by the British experience on the subcontinent, so much so that a consistent pattern of false expectations can be discerned in the colonial reports on approaches that were expected to work in Burma because they had done so in the Madras or Bengal Presidencies. This colonial view that Burma would easily fit into an evolving, generalised picture of British Indian medicine, alongside the region's frontier status, meant that the possibility that its local conditions needed to be taken seriously was overlooked. As we shall see, these assumptions led to disastrous miscalculations on the part of the colonial vaccination staff. For instance, the caste system proved to be a huge obstacle to vaccination in India. Colonial medical authorities hoped that its absence in Burma would mean smooth sailing for the vaccination campaign. Colonial optimism, however, quickly faded when medical officers came up against numerous other unexpected hurdles peculiar to Burma, all of which substantially slowed the progress of the vaccination programme.

While including other areas on British India's periphery in this study was considered, and would perhaps have been wise, they fell outside the writer's linguistic expertise. This mattered because an important concern was to explain how much, or how little, the indigenous population had to say about a development that so intimately affected their lives. This study not only makes extensive use of colonial medical documents on smallpox vaccination in Burma, but also dips into indigenous language texts wherever helpful. In the context of a broader secondary literature on public health in British India emerging, the writer found that though various provincial vaccination departments shared many difficulties in extending operations, there were important differences in how their vaccination programmes progressed.

[2] Mary P. Callahan, *Making Enemies: War and State Building in Burma* (Ithaca and Singapore: Cornell University Press and Singapore University Press, 2004), 21–44.

Situated as it was in a corner of British India, Burma's Vaccination Department was, in many ways, more disadvantaged than those in many provinces on the subcontinent. For one, the transport infrastructure was poorly developed despite the region's importance as an agricultural centre that contributed more to Indian coffers than it received. Limited funding was a continual problem as also the chronic shortage of medical staff. In addition, the vaccination establishment in Burma lacked intra-provincial uniformity because of the administrative separation between Upper Burma and Lower Burma, a fallout of the colonisation process in which Britain extended its rule piecemeal over the region. These disadvantages, however, contributed to the emergence of a vaccine research environment where it was necessary for colonial medical officers to cultivate a detailed understanding of local conditions in their multiple roles as doctors, administrators, and researchers.

## *Vaccination as Medical Technology*

In Burma's colonial administrative culture, the concern for indigenous health was always at the bottom of a pyramid, which had, at its apex, the desire to encourage commercial growth, especially the export of rice. However, smallpox vaccination was given a special place in colonial medicine, and plans to set up a vaccination establishment were on the cards from the early stages of colonisation. David Arnold argues that the East India Company, engaged in establishing itself as the sole authority in an unfamiliar place, sought to make clear the contrast between the violence of its establishment and the promised benevolence of its rule. Vaccination was not introduced with just an enclavist intention, but rather as proof of the company's concern for the well-being of humanity and to demonstrate how advanced European civilisation was.[3] Even

[3] Harrison, *Public Health in British India*, 82; David Arnold, *Colonizing the Body: State Medicine and Epidemic Disease in Nineteenth-Century India* (Berkeley: University of California Press, 1993), 120, 135–36. The East India Company was not exceptional among the European powers in Asia at this time. De Bevoise, for example, explains that the smallpox vaccination programme in the Philippines, begun in 1805, was considered to have been "Spain's finest accomplishment" in the colony, demonstrating Spanish benevolence towards the colonised population. These self-promoting claims were supported by

so, the tendency to minimise administrative costs meant that the medical establishment was always underfunded and understaffed.

Attention to the grand designs and motives of the colonial administration, however, masks many other goals and concerns that complicated the implementation of colonial medical policies. Alongside the growth of the colonial state, the nineteenth century also saw the emergence of modern medicine, with a compelling agenda and notions of being an independent medical agency which had its own peculiar obligations towards the improvement of mankind. As Dorothy and Roy Porter point out, the leaders of the public health service in nineteenth-century Britain "considered themselves to be the embattled vanguard of preventive medicine".[4] While the colonial state saw that the support of preventive medicine could be beneficial to the economy as well as provide a service that was expected of the state, many of its doctors passionately believed they were more than agents of the state. They brought with them from Britain notions of their obligations to the public good. There were thus some colonial medical men who carried out vaccination as a gesture of benevolence.

The colonial government also promoted vaccination because it was a proven Western technology. Albert Fytche, the Chief Commissioner of British Burma, expressed absolute confidence in the superiority of vaccination in his report on the procedure in 1868, advocating the necessity of overcoming Burmese prejudices "by affording them visible and unmistakable proof of the superiority of the vaccine disease, and of its entire freedom from danger".[5] Many colonial medical officers, however, soon realised that vaccination's effectiveness often diminished in tropical environments such

some official reports that indicated the establishment of a well-organised and efficient apparatus led by the Central Board of Vaccination. This included Spanish vaccinators in every provincial centre who instructed hundreds of Filipino vaccinators working in the various pueblos. However, after closer examination, De Bevoise argues that the vaccination programme in the Philippines during the last quarter of the nineteenth century was hardly a success. See Ken de Bevoise, *Agents of Apocalypse: Epidemic Disease in the Colonial Philippines* (Princeton: Princeton University Press, 1995).

4 Dorothy Porter and Roy Porter, "The Politics of Prevention: Anti-Vaccinationism and Public Health in Nineteenth-Century England", *Medical History* 32, 1988, 236.

5 *Report on Vaccination for 1868* (Maulmain: Advertiser Press, 1870), iv.

as Burma because vaccine lymph became effete, or lost its vigour, very quickly, dealing a blow to the superiority of Western medicine. This study identifies the unavailability of effective vaccine lymph as one of the central issues of the smallpox vaccination discourse in colonial Burma and other places in British India. Recent work by Sanjoy Bhattacharya, Mark Harrison, and Michael Worboys on the subject shows that technical questions concerning vaccine lymph played an important role in shaping the vaccination operation in India.[6] While this study finds evidence of the same kind of problems in Burma and on the subcontinent, the chronic lack of effective lymph had a much more significant impact on the vaccination discourse in Burma. At the same time, the ways in which colonial medical officers and researchers in this corner of the empire overcame technical difficulties, provide a useful prism through which to examine the development of colonial medical science and practice.

Understanding colonial medicine and its frequent forays into bacteriology, which were critical for research in lymph preservation, requires an examination of the relationship between the imperial metropole and its colonial periphery. Arnold has pointed out that the historiography of colonial science, technology, and medicine in British India has now transcended the outdated Eurocentric view of a unilateral diffusion of progressive Western "metropolitan" science and practice to passive indigenous recipients in the non-Western world. Instead, historical research on this topic now focuses on the more complicated and dialectic relationship between Western and colonial science. And, "local" knowledge and "local" agents were essential elements in the evolution of colonial science.[7]

Likewise, in colonial Burma, technology transfer in the form of scientific and medical information cannot be viewed as just a binary,

[6] Sanjoy Bhattacharya, Mark Harrison, and Michael Worboys, *Fractured States: Smallpox, Public Health, and Vaccination Policy in British India, 1800–1947* (London: Sangam Books, 2005).

[7] David Arnold, *Science, Technology and Medicine in Colonial India,* New Cambridge History of India (Cambridge: Cambridge University Press, 2000), 9–15. Also, it should not be forgotten that Western "metropolitan" science itself was not a fixed monolithic entity; rather it was "a moving metropolis" of changing places and time. Roy MacLeod, "On Visiting the 'Moving Metropolis' in Reflections on the Architecture of Imperial Science", *Historical Records of Australian Science* 5, 1982, 1–16.

metropole-periphery, relationship. Colonial medicine and science in Burma developed in the context of information networks not confined to flows from the metropole to the colonial periphery. It developed by also drawing on medical and scientific data produced elsewhere in British India and in other European colonies such as British Malaya and the Dutch East Indies. There was thus a multilateral flow of information about new medical techniques and the outcome of scientific research on the cultivation of vaccine lymph in a tropical environment. It is more accurate to view the arena of medical research as a politically undifferentiated landscape across tropical Asia (and even Africa), dotted by a network of vaccine institutes and depots that moved information on their experiments and discoveries regardless of their administrative position within different and competing colonial states. Colonial medical officers at different depots in Burma were not passive recipients of information flowing from London, Calcutta, or Madras, but active contributors to an emerging international discourse on the cultivation and preservation of vaccine lymph. They conducted various experiments, tested out new techniques, designed and used new medical equipment, and mobilised data on Burma's peculiar climatic conditions that affected the vitality of vaccine lymph.

The ways in which colonial medical officers experimented with various medical techniques in an effort to identify the one best suited to local conditions also raises important questions concerning the intersection of local knowledge and colonial science. Deepak Kumar identifies an interest in, and respect for, "local" knowledge among colonial civil officials in British India when it came to the "natural history" of local areas and the "social ecology of the society". Nevertheless, he finds that local knowledge was not crucial for "the technical experts who were products of a 'technical discourse' of science, and who used certain universal parameters to which the local variation had either to conform or get rejected".[8] This study will examine the ways in which the colonial medical men deployed their "local" knowledge of Burma—its climate, topography, animals, markets, transportation difficulties, and indigenous culture—in the effort to cultivate effective vaccine lymph.

[8] Deepak Kumar, *Science and the Raj, 1857–1905* (Delhi: Oxford University Press, 1997), 231.

## *The Rationality of Indigenous Resistance*

Another major theme is the nature of indigenous resistance. There was a difference between the problems faced by the colonial authorities in British India generally and in Burma specifically. Resistance to vaccination was certainly not by any means anti-colonial and Peter Baldwin, Nadja Durbach, and other scholars have drawn attention to the fact that compulsory vaccination was resisted in metropole Britain and Europe just as fiercely as it was on the subcontinent.[9] In British India, Bhattacharya, Harrison, and Worboys suggest, it was a great fear of post-vaccination reactions, which could turn dangerous, that was behind strong indigenous resistance to compulsory vaccination.[10] Burmese parents also had this fear and, like Indian parents, it discouraged them from getting their children vaccinated. However, there were some significant differences between the situation on the subcontinent (as well as in Europe) and Burma, not in the scale of resistance, but in its quality. On the subcontinent, for example, there was a diverse but clear discourse that colonial medical authorities found easy to classify as religious and cultural in nature. Resistance to vaccination could be attributed to caste and notions about polluting the blood or to the importance of the cow, and concern about the pain undergone by the animal in the process of cultivating lymph. However much the colonial medical authorities regarded these views as backward, they could at least easily identify them. In contrast, the resistance in Burma did not fit the prevailing taxonomy. The absence of caste and a weaker understanding of Burmese culture and society meant that the explanations for resistance in India offered no clue. The colonial medical establishment in Burma remained confused about why there was continuing indigenous resistance to vaccination. To complicate matters, it appeared more ambiguous, milder, and more apathetic than that on the subcontinent, making it more difficult to confront or resolve.

[9] Peter Baldwin, *Contagion and the State in Europe, 1830–1930* (Cambridge: Cambridge University Press, 2005); Nadja Durbach, *Bodily Matter: The Anti-Vaccination Movement in England, 1853–1907* (Durham and London: Duke University Press, 2005); Porter and Porter, "The Politics of Prevention", 231–52.

[10] Bhattacharya, Harrison, and Worboys, *Fractured States*, 235–36.

The prevailing literature on indigenous resistance is dominated by generalisations developed to explain the phenomenon in British India, but they are of little help in understanding the Burmese situation. For instance, Arnold looks at the indigenous preference for variolation, or inoculation, in India to explain why there was a resistance to vaccination. He offers the "raw secularity" theory, which says that Indians conceptualised smallpox as a manifestation of the Hindu goddess Sitala and did not want a medicine or a medical practice, such as vaccination, which had the potential to fuel her anger. Rather, they wanted a ritual to sedate her wrath. To meet this need, indigenous variolators called *tikadars* (mark-makers) presented their operations as religious ceremonies.[11] Similarly, Harish Naraindas' argument that it was the therapeutic nature of inoculation, which involved careful dietary instructions and personal attendance on the patient, that encouraged a preference for it over vaccination in India, has only limited relevance to Burma.[12] Other commonly cited cultural and religious factors, such as caste, also do not apply to Burma. So other explanations are necessary to account for the scale and strength of the Burmese resistance to vaccination during the colonial period.

In the Burmese case, the colonial medical authorities simply ascribed the preference for inoculation to what was perceived to be its place in traditional culture. Though colonial medical officers saw it as the major reason for the slow progress of vaccination, their reports are, with the exception of a few vague references, strangely silent about Burmese inoculation methods until 1912. In that year, R. S. Castor published an article in *The Journal of Tropical Medicine and Hygiene* describing Burmese inoculation techniques in detail. Unfortunately, indigenous medical texts are also silent on the subject of inoculation, making corroboration of Castor's description

[11] Arnold, *Colonizing the Body*, 122–33; Similarly Peter Boomgaard, in examining colonial vaccination policies and practices in the Dutch East Indies, argues that the belief that vaccination was against the "will of God" discouraged many outer islanders (that is, non-Javanese Indonesians) from submitting to it. See Peter Boomgaard, "Smallpox, Vaccination, and the Pax Neerlandica Indonesia, 1550–1930", *Bijdragen tot de Taal, Land-en Volkenkunds* 154, no. 4, 2003, 590–617.

[12] Harish Naraindas, "Care, Welfare, and Treason: The Advent of Vaccination in the Nineteenth Century", *Contributions to Indian Sociology,* n.s., vol. 32, no. 1, 1998, 67–98.

difficult. Nevertheless, Burmese inoculation methods appear to have been very close to the techniques used in tattooing—the same tools were used, and the same agents (tattooists and traditional medical practitioners) were involved in both procedures. This raises the issue of socialisation, where the Burmese may have continued to rely on inoculation because it was already an intimate part of the social landscape, whereas both vaccination and vaccinators were foreign. The "traditional" place of inoculation in Burmese society, however, should not be overemphasised. Although smallpox was a periodic scourge in the country since the first recorded outbreak in 1367,[13] the adoption of inoculation is conventionally attributed to the end of the eighteenth century, when Burma annexed the Arakan region on the frontiers of Bengal and deportees to the capital imported the practice of inoculation. There was a rational basis for the adoption of this practice and the indigenous preference for it,

13 Historical documentation of smallpox in Burma is difficult to find before the British arrival except for a few short notes and vague reports made by European travellers and early missionaries. Burmese sources such as chronicles occasionally mention smallpox in the context of royal deaths, but tell us little about the malady outside court circles. The earliest recorded incidence of smallpox in Burma occurred in 1367 when a Burmese king died from the disease. *Hman-nan maha-ya-zawin-daw-gyi* (Yangon, 1967), 1:400. By the eighteenth century, a picture begins to emerge that smallpox became a bigger problem during periods of military campaigning, when Burmese armies moved through wide expanses of territory and presumably encountered populations suffering from the disease. When King Taninganwei (1714–1733) led his army against Gharib Newaz of Manipur, for example, smallpox decimated the force after they reached the Chindwin river. Victor Lieberman, *Burmese Administrative Cycle: Anarchy and Conquest, c. 1580–1760* (Princeton: Princeton University Press, 1984), 210. King Alaunghpaya (r. 1752–1760), the warrior who founded the Konbaung Dynasty (1752–1885), was also reported to have been a victim of smallpox. Europeans noted smallpox cases in Burma, at least from the early eighteenth century. Alexander Hamilton, for example, recorded smallpox in Pegu about 1709, writing that smallpox was "dreaded as pestiferous", and that the neighbours of the stricken would flee two or three miles as soon as anyone caught it. As Hamilton also observed in 1727, a smallpox victim was left with "a jar of water, a basket of raw rice, and some earthen pots to boyl it in, then they (neighbours) bid him farewell for twenty-one days". Alexander Hamilton, *A New Account of the East Indies* (London: Argonaut Press, 1930), 2: 33. The actual magnitude of smallpox epidemics in Burma did not become clear, however, until colonial doctors began to compile statistics on local deaths and diseases under British rule.

for the Burmese were as concerned about the potential dangers of vaccination as the Indians discussed by Bhattacharya, Harrison, and Worboys.

## *Imperial State Medicine*

The main focus of this study is the colonial medical establishment in what was the British province of Burma, not the indigenous population. The most crucial part of the medical experience in colonial Burma was the introduction of imperial state medicine, in particular the establishment of a Vaccination Department to combat disorganised, rural-based, autonomous indigenous practices. At first glance, this would seem to suggest that the Vaccination Department had an easy time in getting the population to accept vaccination. Despite the appearance of uniformity and centralisation, an image fostered by official vaccination reports, the colonial vaccination establishment was in reality rather decentralised, with colonial medical officers fighting among themselves as much as against the indigenous population.

Further, recent literature has shown that indigenous medicine and medical knowledge were not as monolithic and static as they are sometimes made to appear in the older sources. The contributors to Charles Leslie's volume on the plural medical systems of "non-Western" medicine in Asia, for example, show that indigenous medical systems were always evolving, and that they were not simple or unscientific systems.[14] Various indigenous medical systems and beliefs continuously diffused their practices and competed with each other. Hartmut O. Rotermund, for example, examines Edo Japan's multiple local interpretations of smallpox. Some viewed the disease as supernatural in origin and sought cures in spells, while others understood it to be a contagious disease that required a medical solution.[15] At the same time, as Waltraud Ernst explains, there is a risk in categorising "non-Western" medicine or medical systems in false dichotomies. In such a view, she observes, Western

[14] Charles Leslie, ed., *Asian Medical Systems: A Comparative Study* (Berkeley: University of California Press, 1976).

[15] Hartmut O. Rotermund, "Demonic Affliction or Contagious Disease? Changing Perceptions of Smallpox in the Late Edo Period", *Japanese Journal of Religious Studies* 28, nos. 3–4, 2001, 373–98.

medicine is perceived as scientific, and since non-Western medicine is its binary opposite, it is taken to be completely unscientific.[16] This creates an artificial and inaccurate framework, lacking the potential for nuance. Such a preconceived model of "indigenous medicine" might lead to the wrong assumption that the specific system of indigenous medicine before one includes characteristics, principles and practices that it really does not, and vice versa.

An examination of the ways in which British medical men observed Burmese indigenous medicine makes it difficult not to view it as a "dichotomously arranged category". Burmese *hse hsayas* (indigenous medical practitioners) themselves, however, contributed to this mode of characterisation by operating within a shroud of secrecy, closely guarding their medical treatments and treating patients covertly, something they are inclined to do even today.[17] In the case of indigenous treatments for smallpox, they kept their methods just as secret.[18] Thus, the disorganised autonomous nature of indigenous medical practices, deeply rooted in indigenous society and culture, meant that they could not be defeated easily. There was no corpus of indigenous inoculation literature to disprove. There was no single group of medical doctors or a prominent social class to displace. While there was a colonial discourse among colonial medical officers, there was hardly a dialogue between them and the indigenous population.[19]

16 Waltraud Ernst, "Plural Medicine, Tradition and Modernity: Historical and Contemporary Perspectives: Views from Below and from Above", in *Plural Medicine, Tradition and Modernity, 1800–2000*, ed. Waltraud Ernst (London and New York: Routledge, 2002), 2–3.

17 Keiko Tosa, "Weiza Beliefs and Healing: Rituals for the Prevention of Disease and Disaster", paper presented at Burma Studies Conference 2006. The writer is grateful to Professor Tosa for sharing her paper.

18 Sein Khwe, "Kyauk yoga: kagwe-ye hnin kudanyi" (Smallpox: Prevention and Treatment), in *Thudaw ye daw myanma hse pinya* (Yangon: Pyidu kyanma-ye akyawpyu), 3:43.

19 The failure to communicate with the indigenous population was a problem inherent to colonialism in general. In his examination of American medical and sanitary projects in the Philippines during an outbreak of cholera in 1899–1902, Ray Ileto argues that cultural misunderstanding was a crucial obstacle to the success of these projects. The American medical programme directed against the spread of cholera included quarantining patients and placing suspected carriers in detention camps, the burning of the houses of cholera patients, and the cremation of those who died from the

## *Immigrants and Colonial Health*

Another development that makes the case of colonial Burma more complicated is large-scale, inter-provincial migration and the challenges this posed to the extension of vaccination in the province. As a result of the rapid expansion of Burma's rice export economy and the encouragement of the Indian Government, hundreds of thousands of Indian immigrants flooded into Rangoon, many of them as agricultural labourers. They provided human inputs that diversified Burma's population, but also introduced new health problems that were reportedly peculiar to an immigrant population.[20] Public health intervention measures such as inspections, quarantining of suspect cases, and compulsory vaccination were quickly carried out to meet the perceived health threat. The desperate nature of this response had to do with the colonial government's twin priorities regarding the new immigrant population. First, their presence was desired because of the positive impact they were expected to have on production and colonial commerce. Second, this had to be balanced against the serious outbreaks of contagious diseases such as smallpox and cholera they were said to be responsible for.[21]

On the basis of a detailed demographic study of Burma's colonial period, Judith Richell has recently demonstrated the statistical insignificance of the number of cases of cholera and smallpox

disease. This treatment of cholera, Ileto asserts, was not in agreement with indigenous Filipino understandings that "refused to disassociate the disease from the network of social relationships in which it appeared". Reynaldo C. Ileto, "Cholera and the Origins of the American Sanitary Order in the Philippines", in *Imperial Medicine and Indigenous Societies*, ed. David Arnold, (Manchester and New York: Manchester University Press, 1988), 135.

20 The seasonal character of Indian migration to Burma and Indian immigrant health issues have been recently re-examined. See Amarjit Kaur, "Indian Labour, Labour Standards, and Workers' Health in Burma and Malaya, 1900–1940", *Modern Asian Studies* 40, no. 2, 2006, 425–75.

21 This topic has not been examined extensively with reference to British India, a few studies notwithstanding. Mark Harrison, for example, shows that the quarantine debate in the late nineteenth century was a site of conflicting interests between the imperial metropole and the Government of India over colonial commerce and the government's relationship with the indigenous elites. Harrison, *Public Health in British India*, 117–38.

reportedly brought to Burma by Indian immigrants.[22] However, there were understandable reasons for the concern of the colonial health authorities in Rangoon and other ports in British Burma. One was that the sheer volume of immigration threatened to overwhelm the already overstretched resources of the medical establishment. Another was that the huge numbers could not be accommodated quickly in overcrowded Rangoon. Many of the immigrants were forced to live in crowded, unsanitary, unventilated, and generally abysmal housing such as coolie barracks. One of the biggest concerns was that many of these immigrants were seasonal, making it difficult to register them, a factor that made it hard for port health officers to identify sources of disease outbreaks with any degree of certainty. Finally, there were inter-provincial obstacles to cooperation that would have made it possible to vaccinate all prospective immigrants before they left Indian ports. So Burma saw a vigorous debate over the question whether legislation was necessary to make vaccination compulsory for all immigrants on incoming vessels. Among those participating in the debate were health officers who supported such legislation, and mercantile communities who opposed any measure that would make immigration to Burma less attractive to Indian labour.[23]

This study will suggest that the debate over how to respond to Indian immigration reflected one of the significant themes in the development of the smallpox vaccination establishment in colonial Burma—the emergence of a great divide between urban and rural smallpox control. The desperation over preventing smallpox in Rangoon and the legislation and medical intervention that followed took a different path from that of rural Burma, where many villages and towns remained unfettered by compulsory vaccination laws until the 1920s.

22 Judith L. Richell, *Disease and Demography in Colonial Burma* (Singapore: National University of Singapore Press, 2006), 177–78.

23 The emergence of international sanitary regulations focusing on the reform of quarantining has been examined in relation to international commerce, diplomacy, and mercantile interests by Mark Harrison in "Disease, Diplomacy and International Commerce: The Origins of International Sanitary Regulation in the Nineteenth Century", *Journal of Global History 1*, 2006, 197–217.

### *Structure of the Study*

This study begins in the nineteenth century, when Burma came under British rule after three successive wars, and ends with the province's constitutional separation from India in 1937. The major themes of the vaccination effort are presented in seven chapters. The first three focus on the technological issues concerning the lack of effective vaccine lymph. Chapter One examines the inter-provincial and intra-provincial problems involved in transporting vaccine lymph, and colonial plans to produce lymph locally to overcome these difficulties. Chapter Two examines the establishment of local vaccine depots to raise animal lymph in the province of Burma. Cultivating lymph locally meant expanding the field of information necessary for vaccination operations. Colonial medical officers had to gather a varied range of data, from about the local climate to animal markets, and about different localities in the province to identify a spot to establish a depot that would run efficiently. Chapter Three examines the Meiktila vaccine depot's role in conducting local experiments on the cultivation and preservation of vaccine lymph in a difficult tropical environment. It also highlights the vaccine depot's contributions and debts to an evolving information network that linked vaccine cultivation research across tropical Asia, both in British India and in other colonies such as the Dutch East Indies.

The discussion then shifts to indigenous resistance to colonial vaccination policies and practices, and collaboration with them. The colonial medical establishment in Burma found it was necessary to win the hearts and minds of the indigenous population to the vaccination cause. Propaganda, legislation, vaccinators, and inoculators were central to the outcome of the struggle that followed. Chapter Four examines how and why, in its early years, the colonial vaccination establishment failed in communicating to the people that it had a "superior" method. By focusing on the language qualifications of the colonial medical officers as well as efforts at propaganda supporting vaccination in British Burma, it argues that the British colonial government lacked both the ability and the interest to transmit its medical knowledge to the indigenous population. Chapter Five focuses on indigenous inoculation, something colonial medical officers saw as a major obstacle in the way of vaccination. It examines the inoculation method and its similarity to other local practices, which made it familiar to the indigenous population. It also looks into the problems that were encountered in translating the words "inoculation" and "vaccination" into Burmese, something that contributed to the indigenous confusion about vaccination. The chapter argues that indigenous medical practitioners were not just passive victims of aggressive colonial legislation, but people who quickly figured out how to work the colonial legal system to their own advantage. Chapter Six examines the problems that emerged in the process of indigenising vaccination, which colonial medical officers had hoped would encourage indigenous collaboration. The administrative disorganisation of the Vaccination Department, its lack of funds, the failure of its showcase vaccinator training school in Meiktila, and the unpopularity of vaccinators among the general population contributed to numerous reverses in the effort to develop local cooperation. Chapter Seven looks at the ways in which the colonial government in Burma relied on legislation, compulsion, and prohibition to extend vaccination. As a result of large-scale Indian immigration to Rangoon, tensions emerged among diverse interests, including port and municipal health officers, municipal governments, mercantile communities, and the provincial government, all of which drew the vaccination establishment into territory where it had to tackle new issues and responsibilities.

# 1

# *Transporting Lymph*

Although the medical policies and dominant medical methodologies of British India and metropolitan Britain frequently influenced those of British Burma, conditions in the eastern outpost were different, and local medical officers learnt to cope with the challenges peculiar to the region. When they devoted their attention to identifying the various ways in which the smallpox virus was transmitted in Burma for clues that would help fight it, they began to significantly shape vaccination efforts in the province.

There was also a considerable shift in the way in which colonial doctors in British Burma tackled the problem of ineffective lymph. To demonstrate that vaccination was safe and effective, it was necessary to have good lymph. However, this was usually absent in nineteenth century British Burma, and civil surgeons constantly found themselves using ineffective lymph, which not only made the vaccination operation a failure, but also caused unnecessary pain and abscesses among Burmese children. The problem of ineffective lymph was so acutely felt among British medical officers that some even wondered whether it was worth practising vaccination in Burma at all. So overcoming the problem of obtaining good lymph posed a serious challenge to the Vaccination Department, whose work was already hampered by other problems such as the lack of funds and inadequate staff. We will examine how British medical officers in Burma understood the causes for ineffective lymph, including inter- and intra-provincial transport problems, the ways of transporting vaccine lymph, arm-to-arm vaccination operations, and the incompetence of medical officers within the establishment.

## *Transporting Lymph*

One of the most serious problems the colonial vaccination programme in Burma faced was the failure of vaccine matter such as vaccine lymph and vaccine crusts. The reliance of vaccination (from the Latin *vacca*, meaning cow) on cowpox strains was the major difference between it and inoculation, where the smallpox virus (*variola* or human pox virus) was transferred from one person to another to cause a mild attack of the disease and encourage the body to acquire lasting immunity to it. Some societies with domesticated cattle were aware that there was a relationship between exposure to cowpox and immunity to smallpox. This had been noticed among those who handled cows, especially milkers, and there appears to have been proto-vaccination operations using infected cowpox matter before the late eighteenth century. Nevertheless, it was Britain's Edward Jenner who first committed to writing his success in transferring what was believed to be benign cowpox virus from Sara Nelmes, a milkmaid, to a James Phipps on 14 May 1796, earning him the title "father of vaccination".[1] The reason cowpox was effective for vaccination purposes was that it had "only minor serological differences" from the smallpox virus but the two were "anti-genically related" and cowpox, unlike smallpox, did not have a deadly effect on humans. Instead, the body reacted to the cowpox virus by producing antibodies which could effectively fight smallpox.[2]

Bad vaccine matter, repeatedly referred to with anguish in government vaccinators' reports in colonial Burma, meant vaccine pustules or crusts that lost their vigour during transportation or in storage, before they could be used to infect human subjects to produce a positive response. Vaccination with bad vaccine lymph

[1] There has been some controversy regarding Jenner's initial vaccine, which is now believed not to have been derived from either cowpox or smallpox, but horsepox. Donald R. Hopkins, *The Greatest Killer: Smallpox in History* (Chicago: University of Chicago Press, 2002), 7.

[2] Birendra Nath Ghosh, *A Treatise on Hygiene and Public Health* (Preventive and Social Medicine), 15th ed. (Calcutta: Scientific Publishing Co., 1969), 529; Hopkins, *The Greatest Killer*, 79, 88; Robert F. Kahrs, *Viral Diseases of Cattle*, 2nd ed. (Ames: Iowa State University Press, 2001), 201–202; John H. Dirckx, *Stedman's Concise Medical Dictionary for the Health Professionals*, illustrated 4th ed. (Philadelphia: Lippincott Williams and Wilkins, 2001), 577.

resulted in a large number of pustules all over the body, high fever, and/or "unhealthy ulcers of more or less severity".[3] Obtaining good vaccine matter, which remained vigorous, was a constant concern of government vaccinators in colonial Burma, though strenuous efforts were made to identify both good matter and technique. Howard Malcom, a roving informant for the American Baptist Mission in the mid-nineteenth century, mentioned during his travels through Burma, "Matter has been brought from Bengal, Madras, England, France, and America; put up in every possible mode, but in vain".[4] Lymph that proved effective elsewhere turned inert by the time it reached vaccinators in Burma. British medical officers and vaccinators constantly reported the failure of vaccination because of bad lymph.[5]

The medical establishment in Burma had to concern itself with technical problems such as conveyance. The time required to convey the virus from Europe, or other areas more closely associated with the metropole (such as India), to Burma provided opportunities for natural factors (for example, heat) or human error to damage the lymph. The problem of transporting lymph affected Burma in two different ways. There were problems, within the British Empire, of inter-provincial and intra-provincial transport. Inter-provincial transport involved moving the vaccine virus from its place of origin to Burma, which, as one of the empire's provinces far removed from the European metropole, was disadvantaged by the time required to cover the distance and numerous transhipment points en route. The National Vaccine Establishment in London (established in 1808) or the Royal Dispensary in Edinburgh usually sent supplies of vaccine lymph to vaccination establishments in India such as Simla and

[3] *Report on the Administration of British Burma during 1866–67*, 82 [hereafter *RABB* followed by the year].

[4] Howard Malcom, *Travels in South-Eastern Asia, Embracing Hindustan, Malaya, Siam, and China; With Notices of Numerous Missionary Stations, and a Full Account of the Burman Empire*, 2nd ed. (Boston: Gould, Kendall, and Lincoln, 1839), 1:195–96.

[5] For example, lymph from England failed in 1871–72 and 1876–77; lymph from Brussels failed in 1881–82; lymph from Calcutta failed in 1869–70 and 1874–75; and lymph from Almora failed in 1874–75. *RABB during 1874–75*, 150; *RABB during 1876–77*, 159; *RABB during 1881–82*, 128; *Report on Vaccination in British Burma for 1869–70*, 5–6 [hereafter *RVB* followed by the year]; *RVB for 1871–72*, 3.

Calcutta, and it was sent from these locations to Burma. The delivery of vaccines from Britain to India was irregular and, as Bhattacharya explains, the journey between these two points often damaged the lymph's potency. Harsh climatic conditions were a reason, while there was also the danger of delay because lymph packages could be held up at any stop along British mailing routes.[6]

Vaccine lymph produced in India also presented similar problems when it came to transport. For some time, the British medical authorities in Burma tried vaccines from different areas of India. Vaccine matter from Calcutta, they found, "generally failed". One of the first such experiences occurred when smallpox hit the bazaar in Maulmain in 1835 and government aid was sought. The authorities in Burma contacted the government vaccinator assigned to Fort William (the headquarters of the East India Company in Calcutta) for vaccine matter. Though sent, the matter proved to be ineffective for some inexplicable reason—"from some cause hitherto unexplained it has in every instance totally failed of the proper effect".[7]

In 1837, the problem of obtaining a good supply of lymph led M. F. Anderson, the assistant surgeon in Mergui (Tenasserim province), to see if a local supply could be organised. He faced a difficult situation. Two or three people were dying daily of smallpox in the town and the government-supplied vaccine from India was not working effectively. He therefore produced new vaccine matter from a single pox pustule on the udder of an "otherwise healthy cow". Using the new "cow pox" vaccine matter, from July to November 1837, he vaccinated 584 people in Mergui. According to his data, the 584 vaccinated subjects included three European children, 10 Indo-British children, and 31 Indian convicts. The rest included indigenous Burmese at serious risk of being infected.

> Several natives, both adults and children were vaccinated, when their parents, brothers, sisters, or other relations were suffering from small

[6] Sanjoy Bhattacharya, "Re-devising Jennerian Vaccine?" in *Health, Medicine, and Empire: Perspectives on Colonial India*, ed. Biswamoy Pati and Mark Harrison, (New Delhi: Orient Longman, 2001), 218.

[7] *Selected Correspondence and Letters for the Years 1825–26 to 1842–43 in the Office of the Commissioner, Tenasserim Division* (Rangoon: Office of the Superintendent, Government Printing, Burma, 1929), 134.

pox in the same room with them—others, whose parents or relations had died some days before from the disease.[8]

Anderson found that for the first two months, the number of smallpox cases decreased, and all the individuals in the above-mentioned categories avoided death from the disease. In July and August 1837, many of the subjects developed a large number of pustules and high fever, but all survived. Even at this stage, however, the indigenous population suffered more severely than the others. The indigenous children, for example, developed more pustules than the Indo-European children. In September and October, the non-Burmese were recovering and the "vaccination progressed regularly in one or two pustules on each arm, with scarcely any constitutional disturbance". Among the Burmese, however, the infection continued to get worse, with pustules appearing all over their bodies and higher fevers. Seven Burmese died five or six days after the pustules had disappeared. Anderson attributed six of the deaths to pulmonary disease and speculated that the seventh, a child, had been "treated by some ignorant Burmans for acute dysentery". While the majority of the Burmese seem to have survived, their painful experience and the seven deaths may have made the cure appear worse than the disease.[9] British medical officers stationed in Burma once again resorted to importing vaccine matter from Britain and India.

The frequent failure of vaccine lymph continued to cause civil surgeons in Burma a great deal of anxiety. In 1869, Keith Norman MacDonald, a noted Scottish violinist, composer, and author, who was at that time the civil surgeon in Prome, asked in frustration, "Is there any use in vaccination as practised with the kind of lymph procurable, and if so to what extent?"[10] Alexander John Cowie, the first Sanitary Commissioner for British Burma, commented in 1869, "I only desire that good vaccine lymph may be forwarded and not the filthy spurious virus which had been lately received".[11] The chronic problem of bad vaccine lymph led civil surgeons in

8 *Maulmain Chronicle* (18 November 1837), 127.

9 Ibid., 127–28.

10 *Report on Public Health and Vital Statistics in British Burma for 1869* (Rangoon: Chief Commissioner's Office Press, 1870), appendix, iv–v [hereafter *RPHVS* followed by the year].

11 Ibid., iii.

Burma to seek private supplies of effective lymph. Some British medical authorities, such as H. Godbier, the civil medical officer in Myanaung, were even driven to carry lymph personally to their stations.[12]

## *Child Vaccinifers*

The crude technologies employed in transporting lymph from Rangoon to rural civil stations, and occasionally from Calcutta to Rangoon, were partly responsible for the frequent failures of the lymph. As Arnold points out, the first, and most reliable, method of transport for some time was arm-to-arm, using children as carriers of cowpox. One of the earliest examples in British Burma occurred in 1835. When a supply sent from Calcutta to Maulmain failed, Commissioner E. A. Blundell requested that the government dispatch two or more infected children to Tenasserim to provide a living source of vaccine matter. Using children as carriers, however, did not guarantee a dependable supply of lymph, as Malcom found in the 1840s, when only a few people in Maulmain could be vaccinated from the 15 to 20 cowpox-infected people sent by the East India Company as vaccinifers.[13]

Nevertheless, arm-to-arm was the method relied on by medical officers in Burma for some time. Procuring children for the purpose, however, was a problem for the few army medical officers who had been recently stationed in Burma. They had to worry not only about the health of the local population, but also of the regiments in the area, to which they were attached and to which they owed primary allegiance. Finding children to act as carriers required special relationships with authorities outside the employ of the East India Company, especially those with more than solely administrative or medical relationships with the indigenous population. Superintending Surgeon Forsyth complained in 1854 to Arthur P. Phayre, the Commissioner of Pegu, that vaccination needed to be reintroduced, because all "efforts hitherto made to effect that object have not been successful", but he did not suggest

[12] *RPHVS for 1868*, 202; *RPHVS for 1869*, appendix, viii–ix; *Report on Vaccination for 1867–68* (Rangoon: Rangoon Times Press, 1868), 52.

[13] Arnold, *Colonizing the Body*, 140; *Selected Correspondence and Letters for the Years 1825–26 to 1842–43*, 134; Malcom, *Travels in South-Eastern Asia*, 1: 195–96.

how the overburdened commissioner could obtain children to be used as carriers of the virus.[14] Fortunately for Forsyth (and for Phayre), an American Baptist missionary jumped at the opportunity, paving the way for a long-term pattern of cooperation between the American Baptist Mission in Burma and the government's vaccination project. J. Dawson, a doctor who would later gain notoriety for his efforts to gain exemption from land taxes and even local levies for watchmen through his connections,[15] offered to enlist and accompany children to Bengal in exchange for free passage on government steamers for himself and two unnamed associates, apparently travelling for unrelated purposes. Dawson's plan was to take six Burmese children to Calcutta, infect them with the virus and use them as carriers of the virus back to Rangoon. Phayre recommended the proposal for its convenience (and, one suspects, economy), "It is seldom that the services of a medical man can be procured to have charge of children while conveying vaccine from one place to another as now proposed".[16]

Despite the limited influence missionaries had in lowland Burma, the inroads made by them into the hill areas, made easier by the expansion of the East India Company's rule into Burma, helped make this plan possible. The "Burmese" children proposed were actually Karen, an ethnic group that was the target of sustained, and largely successful, missionary efforts at proselytisation. They apparently were members of Dawson's Christian "flock" and he took them to Calcutta in 1855. They were vaccinated both in Calcutta and on board ship on the return voyage to Rangoon. From late January to

[14] 1/1 (A) Accession no. 97, 1854, File 40, "Introduction of Vaccination into Pegu", Box 1854 (3), Arthur Phayre to the Secretary to the Government of India, Foreign Department, Rangoon, dated 10 November 1854, National Archives of the Union of Myanmar [hereafter NAUM], 1.

[15] 1/1 (A) Accession no. 322, 1857, File 51, "Memorial of Dr Dawson on Behalf of the American Baptist Mission for the Exemption of Land and Houses from Usual Taxes in Rangoon", Box 1857 (3), NAUM, 1–3; 1/1(A) Accession no. 1032, 1867, File 425, "Mr Dawson's Refusal to Pay Night Watch Tax in Maulmain", Box 1867 (9), Letter from R. Macrae, Maulmain, to D. Brown, Commissioner of Tenasserim Division, dated Maulmain, 10 August 1867, NAUM, 4.

[16] 1/1 (A) Accession no. 97, 1854, File 40, "Introduction of Vaccination into Pegu", Box 1854 (3), Arthur Phayre to the Secretary to the Government of India, Foreign Department, Rangoon, dated 10 November 1854, NAUM, 1–2.

the end of February 1855 (and presumably into March), for about six weeks, Rangoon thus had a good supply of vaccine matter. In 1858, another child was vaccinated in Calcutta, and this made it possible for a medical officer to successfully vaccinate 76 Karens and Burmans in Henzada and in Rangoon; the vaccine matter thus produced allowed for 31 more successful vaccinations before it became effete.[17] As will be discussed more fully later, missionary and colonial complicity played an important part in the eventual victory of British vaccination efforts in Burma.

Resistance to using children as carriers, however, grew as the nineteenth century progressed. This was both health-oriented and culture-determined. There were serious medical drawbacks with the arm-to-arm method, and this raised objections in Burma, just as it did in Britain and in India. Problems with the method, such as the risk of infection, were enough to provoke resistance or at least non-cooperation. The possibility of secondary infection through the "arm-to-arm" method prompted vaccination personnel to look for a new method elsewhere in the British Empire. Arm-to-arm vaccination was found to be the culprit in transmitting other infectious viruses, and diseases such as leprosy, syphilis and erysipelas were reportedly passed around by the process. This appears to explain why the Burmese vaccinated in Pyinmana in 1891–92 rendered the vaccination operation useless after it was performed on them. The civil surgeon complained, "The people . . . are adverse to the removal of lymph from the vaccine vesicles, and . . . immediately after the operation they frequently apply medicaments to destroy the vaccine virus".[18] The search for children to function as carriers gradually ceased in response to the growing concern in England and other countries of Europe over the safety of "arm-to-arm" operations.

There were also cultural and social issues specific to each society. In British India, for example, as Arnold points out, the caste system was an obstacle to continuing with the "arm-to-arm" method because parents did not like the idea of the blood of other children mixing with that of their children. This was not true of Burma. But

[17] *Report on the Administration of the Province of Pegu for 1855–56*, 43 [hereafter *RAP* followed by the year]; *RAP for 1858–59*, 600.

[18] *RVB for 1891–92*, 5.

unlike the rest of British India, which had well-established rail and road transport networks, Burma's poor transportation infrastructure and sparse rural habitation made the "arm-to-arm" method of vaccination difficult, to say the least. The vaccinators had to transport vaccinated children from one distant village to another to make sure they would have fresh lymph to vaccinate other children. It was very hard, however, to convince Burmese mothers that their children, as vehicles of vaccine, had to be taken across great distances to other villages. Attempts were made by vaccinators to retain fresh lymph in capillary tubes, but this resulted in repeated failure. When Simla vaccine matter failed in Burma in 1860, the superintending surgeon of Rangoon made arrangements to carry effective vaccine matter to the interior districts using human vaccinifers.[19] Children remained critical to Burma's vaccination efforts well into the 1890s.

Although those in charge of vaccination admitted that bad vaccine lymph was responsible for secondary abscesses and pain in vaccinated children, colonial medical officers found ways to shift the blame to the indigenous population. The main recipients of the blame were parents. In a colony with a rudimentary administrative system, where no state school system had been established, indigenous parents were held responsible for all that their children did. Parents were blamed for not supervising their children properly, sometimes to an unreasonable degree, given that Western sanitary measures had only been recently introduced in a few places alongside other, more physical aspects of "modernisation", such as paved roads and footpaths. Though they were without such things, parents were chastised for allowing their children to play in the dirt, exposing their vaccinated arms to pollution, and reducing the chances of success the vaccine vesicles would have. Allowing their children to sleep on hard mats, although no other form of bedding was widely available, also drew criticism, because this was supposed to have made vesicles break, decreasing the quality of the potential vaccine matter.[20] C. E. Pyster, the civil medical officer in Sandoway, lamented in 1868,

> The children here are very careless and more so the parents, who allow them to destroy the vesicles when developed so that no lymph can be

[19] *RAP for 1859–60*, 35.
[20] *RVB for 1871–72*, 5.

obtained and much less a crust, though instructions on all points are duly given to them.[21]

A further factor was that an unfortunate indigenous misinterpretation of vaccination made Burmese parents reluctant to submit their children to vaccination. Some of the Burmese, civil surgeons reported, believed that vaccination would cause measles. The reason for this, as W. P. Kelly, the Superintendent of Vaccination in Rangoon, found, was that the Burmese misunderstood measles and chickenpox to be variants of smallpox.[22]

## *Towards a Provincial Supply of Lymph*

The emergence of a local distribution centre in Rangoon for the redistribution of lymph to stations in the interior led to new problems as the borders of the East India Company's possessions (which were absorbed by the British crown in 1858 after the Indian Mutiny), and its vaccination efforts, expanded into the Burmese hinterland. Despite British confidence that the health problems of the indigenous population could be tackled, the prevention of smallpox continued to evade them. The problem of ineffective lymph continued to plague government vaccination efforts, all of which failed during the first few years of the British occupying Rangoon (following the 1852 war). In 1857–58, it was admitted that vaccination efforts were not any more successful than they had been. H. G. Graham, the Superintending Surgeon of Pegu and later Deputy Inspector General of Hospitals, found that although he had received sufficient vaccine matter for the division's military stations, vaccinations were successful only in Rangoon.[23] As British medical officers increasingly discovered, though lymph could be collected in Rangoon, they faced all kinds of problems in taking it to distant stations in Prome or Toungoo, not to mention Arakan, which had been experienced in transporting lymph from Britain to India and from India to Burma.

Due to the poor transportation infrastructure in the province and the limited number of staff available, British medical officers

21 *Report on Vaccination for 1868*, appendix, ix.
22 *RVB for 1867–68*, 46; *RVB for 1871–72*, 4.
23 *RAP for 1857–58*, 42–43.

in Burma sometimes relied on dried lymph. The prevailing practice of storing lymph for most of the nineteenth century was keeping individual doses on glass slides, ivory points, or on threads. Sealed capillary glass tubes to carry pustules and dried crusts from infected tissue were adopted for transport by sea, but this technique was notoriously faulty in the nineteenth century. Carrying the vaccine virus in the form of dried crusts, pustules, and ivory points in capillary tubes did not protect it against the adverse effects of extreme heat, or prolong its longevity during the long, time-consuming trips into the Burmese interior. In 1855, after Calcutta lymph had been initially successful, Superintending Surgeon Forsyth found that it became totally ineffective after a few weeks. The problem of heat was already known, even with regard to lymph used in Rangoon. E. J. Dickenson, the civil surgeon in Rangoon, found in 1857 that he was only able to vaccinate 100 subjects before the pustules turned ineffective, and blamed the weather for this. The following year, Morton and Rankin, who were doctors in Toungoo and Thayetmyo respectively, also failed to successfully vaccinate using government-supplied lymph. When Cowie attempted to vaccinate 423 subjects in Prome with lymph from Simla in 1860, the effort failed, though it had been successful in 1859. The Simla vaccine matter was even less effective in other Burmese districts, such as Bassein and Henzada, and failed altogether in interior districts such as Tharrawaddy and Toungoo.[24]

Again, Burma's weak transportation infrastructure contributed to the problem of bad lymph. Until railways gradually opened up the province in the latter half of the nineteenth century, people and goods were mostly moved by river steamers, but even these had difficulty accessing shallow branches of the main river systems. The inability to transport lymph quickly troubled vaccinators in distant stations in many ways. The most serious problem was the failure of the lymph while it was en route to the stations because the doctors had to rely on the government postal service to send in requests for lymph and receive shipments of it. When Charles W. E. Foster, the civil surgeon in Mergui, complained about the

[24] Arnold, *Colonizing the Body*, 140; L. H. Collier, "The Preservation of Vaccinia Virus", *Microbiology and Molecular Biology Reviews* 18 (1954), 75; *RAP for 1857–58*, 43–44; *RAP for 1858–59*, 600; *RAP for 1859–60*, 35; *RAP for 1860–61*, 31.

delay in receiving good lymph at his station in 1869, Sanitary Commissioner Cowie observed that the surgeon's problems were a fallout of faulty communication and inconvenient steamer schedules. He explained that communication between Mergui and Rangoon was via the government steamer *Defiance*, which sailed between the two ports once every month. Since this schedule was not coordinated with the date for the monthly shipment of government mail from Rangoon, "opportunities of sending letters and packages are frequently lost, thus a detention of two months at a stretch may occur". Moreover, requests and shipments sent through the post had to take the change of seasons into account. Commenting on Foster's report, Cowie added,

> He [Foster] applied for vaccine lymph in the month of September and did not receive a supply until the 9th of December; tubes and crusts of these prophylactic are not usually received here from the Presidencies earlier than at the end of October, because it has been found utterly useless to perform the operation of vaccination with such lymph in British Burma in the rains—this together with the fact that the Mergui Steamer may have left before the arrival of the Rangoon mail, which is often the case, probably account for the delay or no receipt of virus at Mergui until a late date.[25]

Other factors, beyond the quality of lymph itself, received special attention in the *Administration Report for 1869–70*. These included errors in judgement while choosing between good vaccine and bad vaccine, and inadequate skills among the operators (that is, vaccine lymph was carelessly handled). The continued failure of the lymph led to considerable concern among colonial doctors in Burma, prompting them to point fingers at each other, rather than at the problems caused by the tropical climate.

One example of the problems faced in preparing vaccine in Rangoon occurred in 1869. Sanitary Commissioner Cowie and Henry Summerhayes, who was officiating as the civil surgeon in Rangoon, levelled charges and counter-charges at each other in a series of letters written to higher government authorities. The disagreement was over bad lymph delivered from Rangoon to Prome by two indigenous vaccinators. The vaccinators had brought four glass tubes, all supposedly containing fresh vaccine lymph. When the lymph proved ineffective, Cowie wrote that this was because

25 *RPHVS for 1869*, 139–40.

three of the tubes had not been "sealed at one end". He went on to say "the contents were dry and consisted of purulent matter and were consequently perfectly unfit for use".[26] He disposed of the lymph. The contents of the fourth tube were found to be good. Cowie initially speculated that the reason for this was that it had "evidently been received in Rangoon via Calcutta", implying that the Rangoon depot had done a poor job of preparing the other three tubes.[27]

Summerhayes, who, as the officiating civil surgeon in Rangoon, would have been responsible for the three bad tubes if Cowie's allegation was right, took offence. He wrote a letter ("Regarding a supply of bad lymph") to the Home Department of the Government of India, in which he found fault with Cowie for making a false accusation when he claimed that the fourth tube, the only one that contained good lymph, had been sent from Calcutta via Rangoon. Summerhayes explained that "no vaccine lymph in tubes was received from Calcutta by his Department during the past season",[28] and that his depot had been the source of the good lymph found in the fourth tube. As for the three bad tubes, he said that they too had contained good lymph but, as was evident, they had broken in transit. Cowie then wrote that Summerhayes was now trying to avoid taking responsibility for the lymph that had gone bad.

> Mr Summerhayes' efforts to shield his own Department from blame for forwarding bad vaccine lymph to Prome, by impugning very unguardedly in my opinion, my statement makes it imperative that I should in examining the value of his remarks, maintain my own position.[29]

He also chastised Summerhayes for misreading his initial report. First, he argued, he had not said "one word . . . in the extract about 'broken tubes'", only that the three tubes had not been "sealed at one end". Second, he now provided more details about how the three tubes had looked, which, in his opinion, seemed to indicate they had been prepared in a rather crude manner.

> The three short ones had been slovenly and very imperfectly filled, with dark yellow brown matter. They were dirty looking and the attempt to seal them had been still more carelessly done. The truth is, these tubes

[26] Ibid., appendix, vi.
[27] Ibid.
[28] *RPHVS for 1869*, appendix, x–xiv.
[29] Ibid.

were one and all blackened at both ends as if they had been thrust into the flame of a common tallow candle, and although their mouths at one end had been closed up, at the other they remained open.[30]

In contrast, the longer fourth tube, which one would have thought would be the first to break,

> . . . contained clear and translucent lymph. It was filled, clean and very neatly sealed by a small clear bead of glass at either end, and evidently had been, when contrasted with the others, manipulated by a practised hand.[31]

Cowie did not stop there. He continued to point out other things in Summerhayes' explanation that did not square with his own observations. Of Summerhayes' defence that his department in Rangoon did not receive vaccine lymph in tubes from Calcutta, Cowie was extremely sceptical. He had earlier served as the civil surgeon in Rangoon for five years and remembered that his department had always received vaccine lymph in tubes from the superintendent general of vaccination in Simla, which were sent via Bengal. What he had seen of the fourth tube convinced him that it had been sent in the usual manner from Calcutta to Rangoon, and then forwarded to the station in Prome.

The confrontation illustrates the frequent attempts made by many colonial vaccination authorities to redirect the blame for early lymph failures, and the lack of accountability that prevailed in the vaccine establishment in Burma at the time. That there were numerous, and inconsistent, sources of lymph made it easy for medical authorities to shift blame elsewhere. It also made it hard for their detractors to prove they were dodging responsibility. Medical authorities could often only make accusations based on supposition or circumstantial evidence. Summerhayes, for example, could not remember who actually filled the tubes, which implied that it could have been him, the British doctor in Madras, or virtually anyone involved in the supply of lymph to Burma. Anyone could have been at fault; he simply did not know. He attempted to avoid blame for this by criticising the procedures at the depot, for which he could not be held accountable since he was only officiating as the medical officer in charge. He explained,

30 Ibid., appendix, x.

31 Ibid.

> A custom which obtains here of mixing lymph containing tubes received from the Presidencies with tubes filled here appears to me reprehensible as it prevents all comparison of the relative goodness of the lymph procured from different sources.[32]

Cowie, whose zealousness for detail and accountability was so extreme that it drew criticism from his superiors, continued to press the matter. Since Summerhayes could not offer reliable information, Cowie concluded that his opponent had, at the very least, been negligent in supervising the preparation of vaccine lymph in Rangoon, especially since he had not seen the tubes in question. Indeed, Cowie reasserted, the explanation for the one good tube of lymph had to be that it, alone among the four tubes, had been sent from India. Cowie seems to have won the argument, for the correspondence on the matter does not continue. But the exchange raised important questions about the vaccine establishment in Burma. The controversy had occurred at a time when the government was considering a plan to establish a special vaccine department. Seeing that the state of the vaccine establishment in Burma could only be described as premature, Cowie suggested a halt to the custom of medical stations in Burma using vaccine lymph delivered from India and mixed in Rangoon. Instead, he suggested that these stations rely on lymph sent directly to them from the presidencies until efficient staff could be appointed at the Rangoon depot. Others shared similar opinions.[33] In 1868, the deputy commissioner in Sandoway (Arakan district) reported ineffective vaccine, hinting that his hope was for lymph sent directly from England or Simla. Some medical officers in Burma even urged that the practice of using stored lymph be abandoned altogether. For example, Sub-assistant Surgeon and Superintendent of Vaccination Denonath Doss said,

> In vain did I say that to vaccinate children [with] fresh lymph taken from a successful case, from the 6th to the 8th days counting from the day on which the insertion of the virus was made, is much more certain of success than when the operation is performed with dry crusts or lymph in tubes, which often lose their power by heat, exposure, and during their transit to this distant place.[34]

32 Ibid.

33 Ibid.

34 *Report on Vaccination for 1868*, appendix, ii, iv–v.

To reduce the rate of unsuccessful operations at critical times, the colonial government provided new glass capillary tubes and ivory points to each station. But this was not considered sufficient and calls were made for the establishment of vaccine depots in outlying areas of British Burma so that the local medical authorities would not have to depend on external sources (either from India or from Rangoon) for vaccine matter. These calls took into consideration the adverse effects of tropical heat on lymph. One early suggestion, made in 1868, was that a vaccine depot be established in Prome because it had a dry climate, compared to other towns in British Burma (Upper Burma had not yet been annexed), making it an ideal place for producing vaccine. When the plea for the establishment of a depot at a location other than Rangoon was eventually made in 1869–70, it was suggested that it be built independent of a hospital or dispensary. The reason was connected to the difficulty of getting children to act as carriers of the cowpox virus. The underlying logic was that the parents of children from whom vaccinators would be able to obtain fresh lymph would not agree to bring their wards to a place where they "had to mingle with persons seeking assistance".[35] In other words, if a depot was in any way connected with the presence of sick people, the child-carriers of vaccine matter would disappear.

## *Railways in Burma*

One of the major difficulties in the way of successful distribution of even lymph cultivated within the province was that it quite frequently deteriorated during journeys across long distances.[36] When the British began to annex parts of Burma at the end of the First Anglo-Burmese War (1824–26), they found that the existing road networks were rudimentary, and accessing large areas of the region overland was very difficult. At that time, the Irrawaddy, Salween, Sittang, and Chindwin rivers were the main lines of communication and internal trade. This began to change with the gradual expansion of the colonial railway network later in the

35 *Report on Vaccination in British Burma for the year ending 31st December 1868* (Rangoon: Central Gaol Press, 1870), 18; *RVB for 1869–70*, 7.

36 *Triennial Report on Vaccination in Burma for the Years 1902–03 to 1904–05*, 4 *[hereafter TRVB followed by the years]*.

nineteenth century. However, decreasing the time it would take for vaccine to be transported through the province was not the reason the British opted to build railways. It was more the Indian Mutiny and the possibility of easing military operations that motivated the Government of India to construct railways. The construction of the railway network in Burma was subject to considerable delay and its execution was poor, at least in comparison to India, even at the end of colonial rule. Inadequate information and the constraints of the colonial budget, as Maung Shein explains, were responsible for the delay. Most of the planned railway lines in Burma, for example, had to be built in virgin territory, areas which the colonial government lacked information about. More importantly, the colonial government was very reluctant to sanction the construction of railway lines until they had the potential to yield substantial revenues.[37]

The colonial railway project did not begin until 1874 in Prome. The line between Rangoon and Prome, covering 161 miles (259 kilometres), was completed in 1877 and the line from Rangoon to Toungoo followed in 1885. After the seizure of Upper Burma in 1886, the British began to build a railway line from Rangoon to Mandalay and finished it by 1888. Railway mileage expanded to just over 886 miles (1,425 km) from 1877 to 1896.[38] The railway was then extended to Myitkyina on the Chinese border in 1898, and Lashio in 1902. The private Burma Railways Company purchased the lease of the state railways in 1896, and the railway project continued opening lines to Bassein in 1902, and to Maulmain in 1907. With the opening of the railway line in Maulmain, "one could travel across Lower Burma from east to west by land without having to force a way by footpaths and ford innumerable creeks".[39] However, in reality, the railway lines extended vertically

[37] J. S. Furnivall, *Colonial Policy and Practice: A Comparative Study of Burma and Netherlands India*. (Cambridge: Cambridge University Press, 1948), 78; Maung Shein, "State Investment in Burma Railways, 1874–1914", *Journal of the Burma Research Society* 44, no. 2, December, 1961, 169.

[38] Thant Myint–U, *The Making of Modern Burma* (Cambridge: Cambridge University Press, 2001), 223; Josef Silverstein, "Politics and Railroads in Burma and India", *Journal of the Burma Research Society* 45, no. 1, June, 1962, 80.

[39] Furnivall, *Colonial Policy and Practice*, 78.

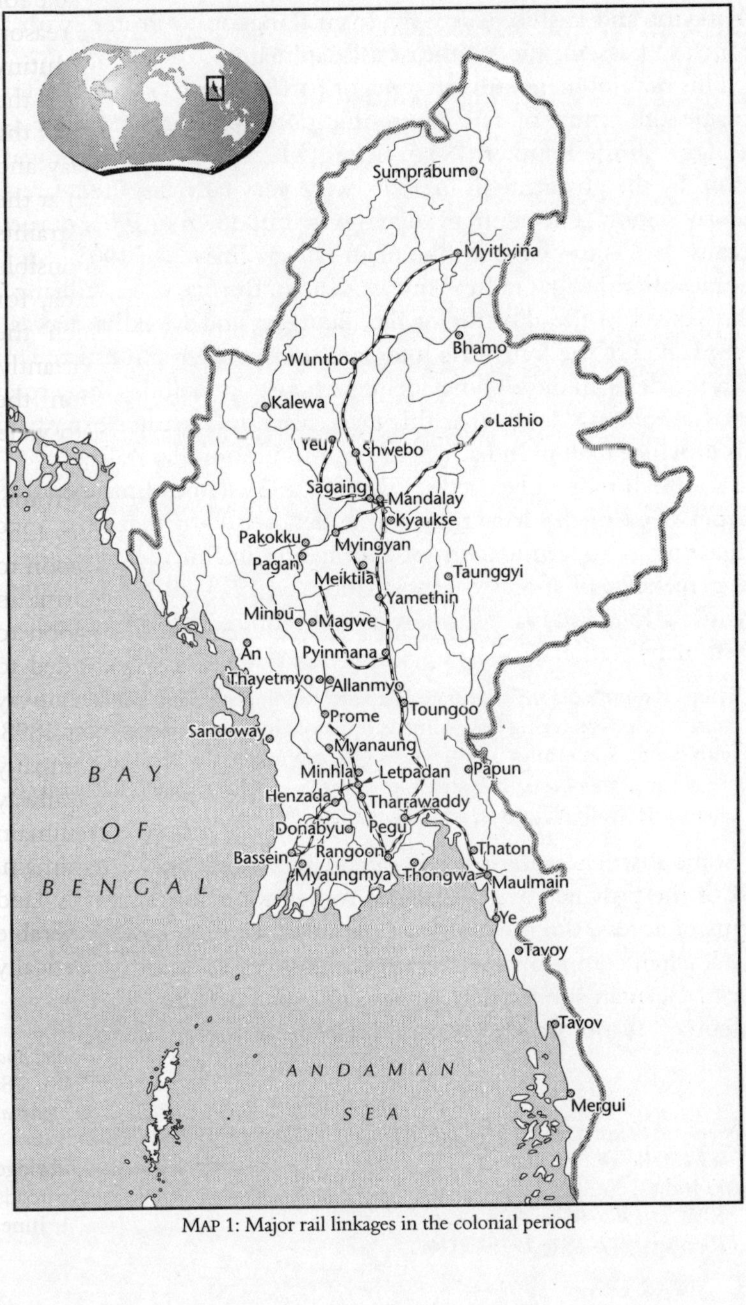


MAP 1: Major rail linkages in the colonial period

from Rangoon to Mandalay; to the northeast in the direction of Myitkyina and Lashio; westward from Rangoon to Prome, with a branch to Bassein; and southeast to Maulmain.

This development still left a major part of Burma's vast interior outside the ambit of rail communication. Some towns such as Taunggyi in the Southern Shan States, where a vaccine depot was set up by the government in 1896, were very far from the nearest railway station. The Taunggyi depot was shut down in 1901, in part because it was too far from the main railway lines.[40] In 1908, three decades after the first railway line was laid in Burma, C. E. Williams, who served as the director of the Taunggyi and Meiktila depots, complained of the long time it took to transport lymph. Frustrated with the delay in developing adequate transport facilities, he wrote that "there is no doubt that this takes place to a greater extent in this province than in India, where communications by rail and road are so much more advanced".[41] Even in 1921, James Entrican, the former head of the Meiktila vaccine depot who at that time was officiating as Superintendent of Vaccination in Burma, considered the percentage of successful vaccinations in 1919–20 "a fair result" because a long interval of time was still required for the lymph to reach many stations.

> I hope it represents the true state of affairs, but in pessimistic moments I cannot help wondering how some vaccinators in far away lonely places, with lymph sometimes 3 or 4 weeks old, can get just as good results as are got in Rangoon or Meiktila, the two places where lymph is always obtainable, fresh, vigorous, and newly made.[42]

Some districts were more isolated. Arakan, separated from the rest of the province by the Arakan Yoma mountain range, was, in terms of access, the most remote region in Burma. During World War I, when communication from Rangoon by sea was reduced for fear of German submarines, it was only approachable overland via Calcutta.[43] It took at least two to three weeks for vaccinators there

[40] *Notes and Statistics on Vaccination in Burma for the Year 1899–1900*, 91 [hereafter *NSVB* followed by the year]; Silverstein, "Politics and Railroads in Burma and India", 80.

[41] *TRVB for 1905–06 to 1907–08*, 6.

[42] *TRVB for 1917–18 to 1919–20*, 4.

[43] Ibid.

to obtain lymph and, generally, Arakan lagged behind other districts in Burma in terms of successful vaccination results.

## *Conclusion*

Late nineteenth century medical reports reveal the frustration and anxiety produced by the failure of vaccine lymph, which posed a seemingly insurmountable problem. Without effective lymph, British medical officers lacked the means to demonstrate that vaccination was a safe and effective method "modern" medicine had come up with. Although "bad lymph" was an easy target for blame, understanding why the lymph failed was a more vexing issue. It revealed the fundamental problems that dogged the effort of building a colonial state in Burma, particularly the lack of personnel and finance, and inadequate infrastructure. Among the causes identified were transportation, the tropical heat, the lack of skilled medical officers, and the irresponsible behaviour of Burmese parents. Transportation delays were due to external factors, such as the time it took to deliver lymph from Britain to India and from India to Burma, as well as internal factors such as the limited reach of Burma's railways and roads. As days went by ferrying the lymph, the heat damaged it. Although the internal transportation system improved, it did not erase the rural-urban divide, and civil surgeons were reluctant to move too far away from the rail tracks. Burmese parents were also blamed for being uncooperative and refusing to allow their children to be used as vaccinifers for arm-to-arm vaccination. This was a serious problem because children were needed to maintain a fresh supply of lymph and also because it showed British medical officers how hollow their hope of an easy vaccination campaign in Burma had been. Unable to point a finger at caste, which was the bugbear in India, British medical authorities took to blaming Burmese "ignorance" and "apathy".[44] This view would largely remain unchanged until the end of colonial rule.

[44] Henry Wells, the Superintendent of Vaccination in Maulmain stated, "In India, where caste is said to be a formidable barrier to vaccination, the Government might hesitate to enforce it; but here, in Burma, we have no such opposing influence, except that arise from ignorance and apathy". *Report on Vaccination for 1868*, appendix, xxix.

# 2

# *Animals and Vaccination*

In 1880, the provincial authorities were still unsatisfied with the progress of the vaccination programme in Burma. In that year, only 51,106 vaccinations were carried out, of which 40,227 were reported to be successful.[1] However, according to the provincial government, four times this number of successful operations was needed to protect the population from smallpox.[2] Colonial medical officers held that both problems, the low number of operations and the high failure rate, were due in part to the same cause, a scarcity of effective lymph. Nonetheless some sanitary commissioners believed that civil surgeons could have overcome the difficulty of obtaining fresh lymph if they had taken a greater interest in their work.[3] Since reliance on ineffective lymph brought from India or Europe via India remained the main cause of unsuccessful vaccinations during the nineteenth century, many civil surgeons in Burma began to recommend that the government set up vaccine depots in the colony for the local cultivation of vaccine lymph.

The calls for lymph cultivation in Burma coincided with the shift from arm-to-arm to calf-to-arm vaccination and to the production of animal lymph at vaccine depots. To pursue the latter course, the vaccination establishment began looking for a suitable location, an area that promised a reliable and constant supply of healthy calves. In the process, civil surgeons paid close attention to Burma's topography, which had earlier not been a major concern of the Vaccination Department. Simultaneously, they renewed their interest in Burma's climate, temperature, and humidity, with special attention to variations in these factors in different areas of

[1] This success rate was far better than that on the subcontinent. Sanjoy Bhattacharya, face-to-face conversation with the author, June 2007.

[2] *RABB during 1881–82, 128.*

[3] *RABB during 1878–79*, 81.

the colony. After the search for a location appeared to be over, the establishment faced new challenges because it now had to act not only as a depot, but also a cattle hospital. It had to have all that was necessary for maintaining cattle health, including proper diets and hygiene, and facilities to treat cattle diseases. Thus developing a serious interest in the health of cattle became vital to the success of the vaccination depot.

## *Calf-to-Arm Vaccination*

Towards the end of the nineteenth century, there was a gradual shift to calf-to-arm vaccination using animal lymph in British India, a change that mirrored what was taking place in Britain and other areas of Europe after concern over the safety of arm-to-arm vaccination had increased. Parents, worried about secondary infections in their children, especially syphilis and leprosy, pressed for an alternative to the arm-to-arm method. In other words, they were against humanised lymph. In the colonies, British doctors already knew there was the danger of transmitting infectious diseases through arm-to-arm vaccination from their experiences at home, for smallpox was not simply a "tropical disease", but a universal malady. In Britain and other parts of Europe, growing concerns over the safety of arm-to-arm vaccination pressured the medical authorities to search for a better method of transferring and preserving good vaccine lymph. Using calves presented a way out. Since the lymph available from cow-to-arm vaccination was fresh and thus more effective and less dangerous, this method spread throughout Europe by the mid-nineteenth century.[4] The European solution thus replaced the child as a carrier of lymph with the cow. Instead of passing vaccine lymph from arm to arm among children, British medical authorities began to inoculate calves with cowpox, other animal poxes or even human smallpox matter. They took the infected calves to patients' doorsteps, vaccinating people directly from the cattle before better preservatives became available. According to Hopkins, this method was first perfected in Naples in 1843, and then adopted in France in 1864, Germany in 1865, and Britain in 1881. Experiments with animal lymph had been successfully conducted much earlier in both British India (1832)

[4] Hopkins, *The Greatest Killer*, 88.

and Tenasserim (1837) to solve the basic problem of obtaining effective lymph. Despite the early successes, it was not until 1880 that experiments in Madras succeeded in producing calf lymph that was reliable enough to make calf-to-arm vaccination an alternative to arm-to-arm vaccination in India. Immediately after this, a supply of animal lymph was sent from the Bombay vaccine depot to Burma as part of a trial.[5]

Burma had launched its own experiments in cultivating animal lymph in the early 1880s, but soon realised that satisfying all the requirements was hard. However, from 1884, more positive reports emerged. Thomas Franklin Pedley, the Health Officer of the Rangoon municipality (1883–90), successfully cultivated animal vaccine, and using the calf-to-arm method, vaccinated 26,000 people around Rangoon.[6] From 1888 to 1890, Pedley personally inoculated more than 456 calves and sent out 1,073 tubes of lymph to other practitioners and vaccinators, even to some beyond the municipal limits. This was a landmark event, which drew praise from his colleagues. Experiments were carried out in other vaccine stations as well. Oswald Baker, the civil surgeon in Akyab, was successful in producing lymph at his station in 1883–84. G. T. Thomas in Maulmain was also successful in inoculating a calf when fresh lymph was needed.[7] However, these efforts occurred on a much smaller scale than at the Rangoon depot.

In 1889, the Government of India communicated "confidential reasons" to Rangoon and other provincial governments about why arm-to-arm vaccination and the use of humanised lymph were being abandoned. Animal vaccination gradually began to replace arm-to-arm vaccination whenever and wherever animal lymph was

[5] Ibid, 88–89; *Maulmain Chronicle*, 18 November 1837, 127; Bhattacharya, "Re-devising Jennerian Vaccine?" 223; Arnold, *Colonizing the Body*, 140; Harrison, *Public Health in British India*, 85, and on 267, citing James, *Smallpox and Vaccination*, 32; *RABB during 1881–82*, 128.

[6] According to one source, "No fewer than 32,742 vaccinations were performed in these districts, of which number 10,484 primary vaccinations and 15,779 revaccinations were successful. The percentage of successful vaccinations for the province amounted to 86.1 for primary cases and 69.73 for revaccination. The latter result is considerably better than that obtained in 1888". *Rangoon Gazette and Weekly Budget*, 18 July 1890.

[7] Ibid; *RABB during 1882–83*, 143; *RABB during 1883–84*, 88; *RABB during 1884–85*, 66; *RVB for 1889–90*, 5.

available.[8] For example, in Maulmain in 1889, Thomas reported ending arm-to-arm vaccination because of an abundance of animal lymph.[9] By 1902, calf lymph vaccination was being carried out all over Burma, arm-to-arm vaccination only being resorted to when calf lymph was found to be inert.

## *The Emergence of Local Depots*

The short life span of animal lymph and the impracticability of transporting cow vaccinifers overseas meant that the adoption of cow-to-arm vaccination in India and Burma required locally produced animal vaccine lymph. As it was, the late adoption of animal vaccine lymph in Britain had delayed its introduction to the colonies. More obstacles were presented by the climate and cultures of the subcontinent and Burma. The tropical climate had adverse effects on experiments with animal lymph for decades. Even more irksome to some of the medical authorities was what looked like a cultural resistance on the subcontinent to using calf lymph.[10]

Cattle had to be taken directly to those who had to be vaccinated before reliable preservation methods replaced cow-to-arm transfer. In Rangoon, in the early 1890s, for example, Pedley relied on direct vaccination in the area under his charge, taking calves in a covered cart through the streets and out to the rice mills. In rural areas, vaccinators would lead calves from one village to the next, directly vaccinating villagers from them. The difficulties and time involved in doing this persuaded the colonial medical authorities in Burma to think of establishing a central vaccine depot for producing animal vaccine, an idea that had been mooted since the early 1880s. The first step came with sanction for a proposal put forward by Griffith, the civil surgeon in Rangoon. His plan was to set up an establishment in Thayetmyo to supply animal lymph for local

8 According to Bhattacharya, Harrison, and Worboys, the calf-to-arm method did not immediately replace arm-to-arm vaccination and both methods were practised side by side on the subcontinent. *Fractured States*, 40–41.

9 IOR/P/7796, Burma File, 1908, W. G. King to the Secretary to the Government of Burma, 10 January 1908, in Home (Medical) Department, Burma, January 1908, OIOC, 5.

10 David Arnold, "Smallpox and Colonial Medicine in Nineteenth Century India", in *Imperial Medicine and Indigenous Societies*, ed. David Arnold, (Manchester: Manchester University Press, 1988), 53.

needs. However, this attempt failed because fresh lymph brought from Brussels repeatedly lost its efficacy in transit, preventing experiments in lymph cultivation in Thayetmyo. The government later decided to resume the experiments at Thayetmyo by using a supply of animal lymph from the Bombay vaccine depot.[11] While initial attempts failed in Thayetmyo in 1882, the vaccine station in Rangoon was successful, which encouraged the government to think of establishing a vaccine depot there.

In 1889, the Government of India communicated to Rangoon and other provincial governments that henceforth vaccination in British India would rely on supplies of animal lymph obtained by setting up animal lymph depots.[12] Burma already had a working vaccine depot, the Rangoon vaccine depot, which was emerging as a facility capable of supplying animal vaccine throughout Lower Burma. Nevertheless, the Rangoon vaccine depot was under the Rangoon municipality and never provided with the funds it needed to keep pace with the increasing demand for lymph. It failed to convince local business and social leaders on the municipal council, its main source of funds, of the need for more money. The limited funds provided by the council were not sufficient to update its equipment, and the depot's facilities soon became dangerously old and outdated. The quality of the lymph it produced also suffered. Further, as a municipal institution, it was not technically responsible for providing lymph to all places in the province. Through a special arrangement, however, the provincial government paid 850 rupees a year for lymph supplies from Rangoon. The depot therefore provided cultivated vaccine paste gratis to medical officers, sanitary officers, and to public and private vaccinators.[13] The municipality was unhappy with this situation. It resented having

[11] *RABB during 1880–81*, 127; *RABB during 1881–82,* 128; *RVB for 1889–90*, 5.

[12] Bhattacharya, Harrison, and Worboys, *Fractured States*, 188.

[13] IOR/P/7796, Burma File, 1908, W. G. King to the Secretary to the Government of Burma, 10 January 1908, in Home (Medical) Department, Burma, January 1908, OIOC; *TRVB for 1896–97 to 1898–99*, 18; In 1906, King, the Sanitary Commissioner, Inspector-General of Civil Hospitals (Burma), and Superintendent of Vaccination (Burma), was so disgusted by the lack of care for cultivated vaccine lymph in Rangoon that he said he would never use the "vaccine pulp gather[ed] in this depot" under any circumstances. *NSVB for 1905–06*, 2.

to bear some of the cost of supplying fresh lymph to the entire province because the money provided by the provincial government did not cover all its costs. D. Norton and C. R. T. Balston of the municipal council urged, "It would be well if government took over the preparation of lymph for the use of vaccinators throughout the whole of Burma, including Rangoon".[14]

The Vaccination Department decided that it needed its own vaccine lymph depot. Several factors had to be taken into account in the planning of a new central depot. Since the department sought to avoid redundancy, it was decided the depot would be situated further north, in a more central position. Though it was technically possible to cultivate lymph wherever healthy cattle could be found, extremes in temperature and humidity were to be avoided. High temperatures had for long made the cultivation and preservation of lymph in British India more difficult than in Europe. So, across British India, a mild climate became a prerequisite for potential sites of vaccine depots. It was not high temperature that made Rangoon a problematic choice, for Madras, which was viewed as favourable for lymph cultivation, had a higher mean temperature. Instead, what stood in the way was that Rangoon had a very high mean humidity of 78 (Madras had a mean humidity of only 71). Extremely low temperatures, a problem that could be solved by artificial heating, and low humidity would also adversely affect the cultivation of lymph. Thus, in addition to finding a site that was cooler than Rangoon, the Vaccination Department had to find one that was dryer, but not too dry.[15]

Throughout British India, it was found that the best sites were hill stations, located at high elevations with moderate temperatures and humidity. Towards the end of the nineteenth century and into the early twentieth century, a general shift occurred from vaccine depots located only in the major municipalities to additional provincial depots in hill stations such as Bangalore (2,981 feet), Belgaum (2,250 feet), Pachmari (3,528 feet), and Shillong (4,793

[14] IOR/P/6034, File No. 2T–27, Note by D. Norton, CSI, and C.R.T. Balston on the reorganisation of the municipal establishment in Rangoon, Home (Medical), April 1901, OIOC.

[15] *NSVB for 1896–97,* 10; W. G. King, *Vaccination in the Tropics* (London: Tropical Diseases Bureau, 1920), 24; Bhattacharya, Harrison, and Worboys, *Fractured States*, 41–42.

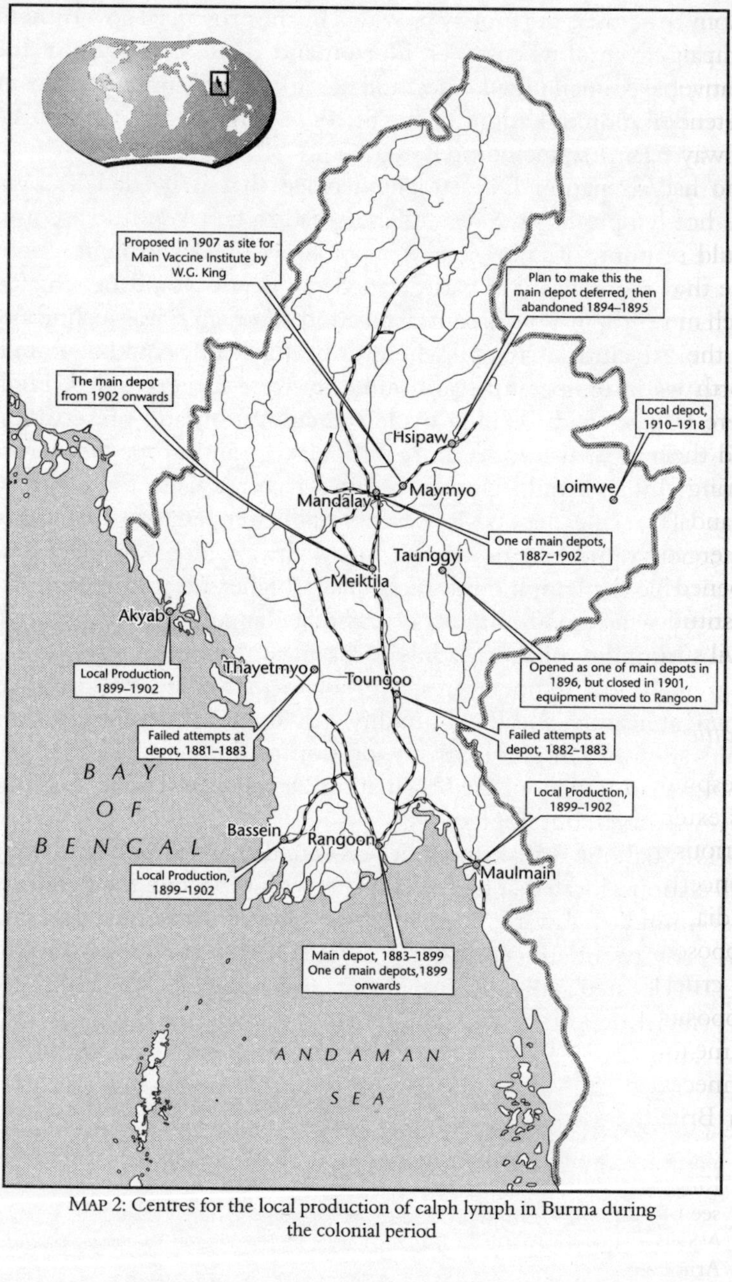


MAP 2: Centres for the local production of calph lymph in Burma during the colonial period

feet).[16] In Burma, similar "ideal" sites became available when the colony's infrastructure was improved after the end of the pacification campaign that had begun in 1886 with the fall of Mandalay. A relatively tranquil countryside untroubled by "dacoit" bands and pretenders to the vacant Burmese throne was now invaded by railway tracks, metalled roads and telegraph lines. British officers, who had been forced to stay close to protected cantonments in the hot lowlands, now sought cool highland retreats where they could settle, bring their families, and live a life that imitated the one they had lived in Britain. Two new hill stations were built for such men in 1896—Maymyo, northeast of Mandalay, and Taunggyi, in the Southern Shan States. Such hill stations in the pacified north were a boon for the Vaccination Department because they were far away from the endemic moisture of the Irrawaddy delta and their elevations offered mild temperatures comparable to the spring in Europe. Of the two hill stations, Maymyo's proximity to Mandalay and the latter's vaccine depot counted against it. Taunggyi emerged as the clear favourite, and the Vaccination Department opened its central depot there in 1896 as "a purely government Institution" under the supervision and management of the local civil surgeon.[17]

## *Cattle Procurement*

Despite the cow-to-arm method's advantages over arm-to-arm, its extension into Burma did not go as smoothly as planned. The serious opposition to the use of cattle as vaccinifers, born of religious concerns, which the Vaccination Department faced in British India, was not there. There, Hindus, especially in Punjab, initially opposed the use of calf lymph because they regarded its cultivation as cruel to the most sacred of animals. According to Arnold, this opposition gradually disappeared, partly because many Indians came to prefer calf lymph to arm-to-arm vaccination, which caused unnecessary pain to children and was generally inconvenient.[18] In Britain, some parents were afraid that their children "might

16 King, *Vaccination in the Tropics*, 24; for other details on these establishments, see Bhattacharya, Harrison, and Worboys, *Fractured States*, 186–87.

17 *NSVB for 1896–97*, 10.

18 Arnold, *Colonizing the Body*, 142.

adopt cow-like tendencies" while others refused to submit their children to vaccination because they believed that the calf lymph would transmit "a nineteenth-century version of mad cow disease". Such concerns were shared and utilised by proponents of the anti-vaccination cause in Britain, who cautioned that animal "vaccination could 'stimulate their animal propensities' and thus 'brutify' and 'lower' human nature".[19] As Baldwin explains, they viewed the mix of human and beast as a violation of nature and as "irreligious, going beyond pollution to abomination".[20] The vaccination establishment still had to solve a number of practical problems such as maintaining a sufficient stock of cattle as vaccinifers so that fresh and effective strains of vaccine lymph could be obtained. Sufficient numbers of calves were necessary for the cultivation of lymph since all the cattle inoculated did not necessarily produce effective lymph. The need to continuously procure enough cattle for the cultivation of calf lymph became an important concern with the emergence of the central vaccine depot in Burma.

Climate was a central factor affecting the supply of healthy calves in Burma. A harsh climate could easily hinder the raising of effective lymph. High temperatures, up to 100 degrees Fahrenheit (38 degrees Celsius) in the hot season, were not uncommon, weakening calves' health. Calves thus enfeebled yielded only a small quantity of lymph with little potency. So the rainy season was the only period when suitable cattle could be acquired.[21] The decision to establish a central vaccine depot in the Taunggyi plateau was intended to offset such constraints, by moving cattle and the cultivation of lymph out of the hot lowlands to the cooler highlands. However, this only replaced one problem with another. Access to water in the highlands was limited, forcing farmers and cattle traders to drive most of their cattle to distant areas that were better supplied. The cattle that remained in Taunggyi were mostly ill and unwanted, and

[19] Nadja Durbach, *Bodily Matters: The Anti-Vaccination Movement in England, 1853–1907* (Durham and London: Duke University Press, 2005), 125–26.

[20] Peter Baldwin, *Contagion and the State in Europe, 1830–1930* (Cambridge: Cambridge University Press, 2005), 285.

[21] "Annual Report on the Working of the Taunggyi Vaccine Depot for 1899–1900", in *NSVB for 1899–1900*, Appendix B, xviii; *NSVB for 1899–1900*, 15, 16.

the depot staff found only cattle in a "wretched" state, unsuitable for the operation.[22]

The importance of cattle to the indigenous people, who were mainly occupied in agriculture, and unpredictable market forces made it difficult for depots running on tight government budgets to maintain a supply of cattle for vaccination purposes. In the early years of a depot's operations, the Burmese could be convinced to volunteer their cattle free of charge. Cattle were only needed temporarily and could be returned to the owner after the depot's use. But the indigenous population eventually began to resist loaning their cows when they realised that the medical authorities were going to infect them. In late 1891, for example, the milkmen and butchers in Thayetmyo refused to allow the vaccination of their calves, fearing they would lose their animals. Usually, however, resistance was not simply based on a fear of losing calves but also on the more justified concern that lesions from the vaccination operation could cause mastitis and lower milk productivity, thus reducing the economic value of the animal. Likewise, there was a belief among local cattle traders that inoculated cows were useless for breeding. Such fears grew worse during bad harvests, when personal economies were at their most precarious. On occasion, the Burmese refused to cooperate because they were dissatisfied with the colonial administration over other issues. In Rangoon in 1890–91, for example, Burmese butchers boycotted the vaccine depot because they were upset by strict slaughterhouse rules and the rejection of unhealthy cattle by the veterinary officer.[23]

Such problems made the depot turn to the purchase system, in which it bought calves from farmers or local markets, and resold them after the vaccine lymph was collected. For the vaccine depot, the major problem with this was the high cost. As early as 1889, the problems involved in acquiring cows had threatened continuing with the cultivation of lymph. In Akyab, in 1890, civil surgeon Evans complained of the high price of animal vaccination, writing that its rising cost outweighed its advantages. The price of a calf at a particular time depended on various factors—agricultural,

22 "Annual Report on the Working of the Taunggyi Vaccine Depot for 1899–1900", xiii.

23 Kahrs, *Viral Diseases of Cattle*, 201; *TRVB for 1905–06 to 1907–08*, 6; *TRVB for 1890–91 to 1892–93*, 9; *TRVB for 1905–1906 to 1907–1908*, 6.

environmental, and climatic. External events sometimes produced adverse market conditions. During World War I, Britain set up prisoner of war camps in Burma for captured Turkish soldiers, who were Muslims and did not eat pork like the Burmese. They had to be fed beef, simultaneously increasing demand for the meat and reducing its supply, which made the price of cattle go through the roof. Vaccine depots also found it difficult to recoup what had been spent on buying cattle because Burmese farmers and butchers were not keen on acquiring inoculated animals. During bad harvests, which were frequent in the 1890s, it was especially difficult to find markets to sell the depot's unwanted cattle.[24]

The hire system, where Burmese suppliers agreed to rent out their cattle for a monetary remuneration, emerged as a partial solution in the late 1890s. Under this arrangement, the Taunggyi (from June 1899) and Rangoon depots hired cattle on contract, and returned them after the vaccine lymph had been collected. Hiring cattle, of course, was more expensive than obtaining the animals at no cost. It was more affordable to do in Taunggyi than in Rangoon. The highest rate paid for a calf in Taunggyi was five rupees in 1899, while in Rangoon, the following year, it was seven rupees. The Taunggyi depot's expenditure doubled in 1899–1900 (about 1,180 rupees) from what it had been in 1897–1898 (about 605 rupees), solely due to the new cattle hiring arrangement. Compared to the purchase system, however, the hiring system was seen as a "financially economical" scheme because hiring cattle was much cheaper than buying them. Since cattle were no longer "owned" throughout the year, they only had to be fed during the time the lymph was cultivated, thus reducing the expenditure on fodder. It was also suggested that the hiring system contributed to a lower mortality rate among the cattle.[25]

Ultimately, the hiring system did little to save the Taunggyi vaccine depot and it closed in June 1901, mainly due to the problems it faced in obtaining calves. To prevent a repeat of this, easy access to cattle became the most important factor in selecting

[24] *NSVB for 1900–1901*, 3; *Report on Vaccination in Burma for the Year 1889–90*, 5 [hereafter also *RVB* followed by the year]; *TRVB for 1905–1906 to 1907–1908*, 6–7; *TRVB for 1917–1918 to 1919–1920*, 4–6.

[25] *NSVB for 1899–1900*, 14, 16; *NSVB for 1900–1901*, 3; *NSVB for 1911–1912*, 4.

Taunggyi's successor. While scouting out a new location, Taunggyi's equipment was sent to the vaccine depot at Rangoon for about eight months. Hopes were entertained that no new move would have to be made if the Rangoon vaccine depot could raise enough lymph to supply all of Burma but an outbreak of cattle disease prevented it from obtaining enough calves for the cultivation of lymph.[26] The proposal to set up a centralised depot for lymph distribution in Upper Burma assumed concrete shape once Meiktila was picked as the best spot to do it in. Meiktila, in the dry zone of central Burma, surrounded by agricultural land, with access to lake and river water, and abundant cattle, had a new depot in February 1902. C. C. Little, the Superintendent General of Vaccination in Burma, explained that Meiktila had advantages over both Rangoon and Taunggyi. Compared to Rangoon, he observed, Meiktila was "cooler and drier",[27] which was better for the efficacy of the lymph. In contrast to Taunggyi, there was ready access to cattle and water, as well as the railway. He said,

> I anticipate no difficulty in procuring suitable calves at Meiktila, as, owing to the presence of a large body of water in the vicinity of this town, droves of cattle during the dry and hot season of the year are brought in from all the villages for miles around and maintained around this lake at distances within easy reach of Meiktila. Arrangements could be entered into for a constant supply of calves, which even should the local supply fail, could be supplemented from adjoining districts by means of the railway.[28]

Although Little believed that at the new location "the supply of calves was not likely to fail",[29] the availability of cattle continued to be a problem for the Meiktila depot, just as it had plagued its predecessors.

Meiktila first adopted the purchase system. This was made easier by cooperation among different government departments to overcome occasional obstacles. When the harvest failed in the area in 1924–25, for instance, and cattle became scarce, Burmese

26 *NSVB for 1900–1901*, 3, 5.

27 *TRVB for 1899–1900 to 1901–1902*, 4.

28 IOR/P/6034 File No. 1Z-5, C. C. Little, to the Secretary to the Government of Burma, 12 January 1901, Home (Sanitary) Department, Burma, February 1901, OIOC.

29 *TRVB for 1899–1900 to 1901–1902*, 4.

township officials accompanied the depot staff when they went to the villages, to help them convince villagers to sell their cattle. The depot staff found this aid crucial in striking deals. The Burma Railways Department also stepped in, and relaxed cattle transport regulations to make it easier for the depot to buy cattle from outside Meiktila district. The Forest Department likewise set up a camp nine miles (14.5 km) from Meiktila in a forest reserve where it gave the depot rights to graze its cattle. To help the depot dispose of older cattle and acquire younger ones, the Forest Department planned to open a market where calves that had reached the age of 18 to 24 months could be sold. Nevertheless, from 1931, the depot reverted to the hire system which had the advantage that the director of the depot could choose healthy calves which were of a suitable age, colour, and size.[30]

## *Ideal Cattle*

The Vaccination Department preferred the use of calves, but also allowed the use of buffalo calves, rabbits, and donkeys if necessary. Young goats could also be used as vaccinifers, but the returns were uncertain. While the buffalo yielded a significant amount of vesicle pulp, it was difficult to keep clean. Experiments in Europe showed the camel was a good vaccinifer and though this was relevant to other parts of British India, it had little to do with Burma, which did not have the animal.[31]

According to the reports of several Superintendent Generals of Vaccination, including Entrican, Williams and Walter Gawen King, certain cattle were better than others for the cultivation of lymph. The preferred cattle had to be about nine months old. Although calves from two to eight months old were used for vaccination purposes in Europe, in India and Burma, calves were only allowed, by "established custom . . . a poor remnant of its mother's milk", which hampered proper physical development in an important phase of life. So, as Entrican pointed out, calves younger than nine months were "too weak and thin" to provide satisfactory

[30] *NSVB for 1924–25*, 8; *TRVB for 1923–24 to 1925–26*, 10–11; *TRVB for 1929–30 to 1931–32*, 12.

[31] J. Entrican, *Notes for the Use of Vaccinators* (Rangoon: Government Press, 1918), 28; King, *Vaccination in the Tropics*, 29f.

vesicles. The depot had to wait until a calf had been weaned before submitting it to the vaccination operation at about nine months of age, although those up to 18 months were also acceptable. Any older, the calf's skin became too tough for a good operation.[32] Calves also had to be of a size that allowed "ready handling and hoisting when placing it upon the operation table".[33] The colour of the calf's skin was also a determining factor though the reasons for this were debated. According to Entrican's 1909 notes, the darker the colour, the tougher the skin would be. Dark-skinned calves were resorted to only if no light-skinned ones were available. "Black calves" were less suitable because the skin of their bellies, aside from being pigmented, was "relatively thicker". King, writing in 1920, also advised that calves with dark pigmented abdomens "should be avoided", though he admitted that the reasons they yielded poor vesicles had yet to be explained. Since it was difficult to tell the colour of the skin from a glance, certain clues were looked for. Williams looked for calves "with red hair and white bellies". Entrican advised that the best way to determine colour was to look at the perineum below the tail, for if it was dark, the skin would also be dark. Finally, the depot staff preferred female to male cattle. Female calves were chosen because they had larger abdomens, which provided a larger surface for vaccination, and were easier to keep clean. On male cattle, "the vaccinated surface and the dressing applied [was liable to] become soiled by urine".[34]

Once healthy calves of the right age, gender, size, and colour were selected, they were divided into two categories, and then physically separated. "Vaccine stock" calves were the "perfect specimens" and had a quiet disposition, making them suitable for the cultivation of seed vaccine. The remaining healthy specimens were the "paste" calves, used to produce the vaccine that would actually be issued from the depot. To keep them separated and prevent mixing them together by mistake, wooden labels with a serial number and the

32 "Annual Report on the Working of the Taunggyi Vaccine Depot for 1899–1900", xv; *NSVB for 1923–24*, 8; Entrican, *Notes for the Use of Vaccinators*, 28; King, *Vaccination in the Tropics*, 29.

33 King, *Vaccination in the Tropics*, 29.

34 "Annual Report on the Working of the Taunggyi Vaccine Depot for 1899–1900", xv; Entrican, *Notes for the Use of Vaccinators*, 28; King, *Vaccination in the Tropics*, 30.

date of admission were attached to their collars. The two groups were separated so that they could be accorded different degrees of care, especially in matters of diet and overall treatment.[35]

## *The Depot and the Cultivation of Calf Lymph*

While preparing for vaccination, cattle hygiene was particularly important. The calf had to be washed thoroughly and kept clean, its hair being brushed every day.[36] Twelve hours before vaccination, the calf was brought to the operation table, which could be tilted both vertically and horizontally by means of hinges. While vertical, the calf was strapped to it before the table was tilted back to a horizontal position. The abdomen was exposed by pulling the calf's legs as far apart as possible, and strapping them down using rope and ring bolts attached to the surface of the table. After the abdomen was washed with warm water and soap to soften the hair, all of it, from the perineum to a point just short of the forelegs, was shaved, care being taken not to break the skin. It was then washed again with soap and sterilised water. The animal was then righted and a "belly apron" tied around its abdomen to prevent contamination by dirt. Twelve hours later, the calf was again put on the table, tied down, and its abdomen washed again. It was then dried with a soft sterilised towel. At no point was antiseptic, particularly perchloride of mercury solution, used because it would interfere with the vaccine. The operation could now begin. The skin of the abdomen was stretched with a finger and thumb and a 3 or 4-inch (7.5 or 10-cm) incision (through the epidermis to the dermis, without puncturing it, so that no blood would be drawn) made with a lancet, followed by parallel incisions between 1.5 and 2 inches apart. Depending of whether glycerinated or lanolinated lymph was used, the person performing the operation would either allow the lymph (glycerinated) to drain off the lancet into the wound, or would make the incisions first and then rub the lymph (lanolinated) into the wound. The whole abdomen was "planted" in this manner.[37]

35 King, *Vaccination in the Tropics*, 30.

36 Entrican, *Notes for the Use of Vaccinators*, 28.

37 Entrican, *Notes for the Use of Vaccinators*, 29–30; King, *Vaccination in the Tropics*, 30–35, 38.

In addition to making sure there was no contamination and physical trauma, the depot was concerned about reducing any psychological trauma the animal might suffer. King suggested that the long time the numerous hygienic steps took actually helped the calf adjust to what might otherwise be a very frightening ordeal. He explained,

> Insistence upon the necessity for gradually making an animal accustomed to its surroundings before inoculation may seem trivial and fanciful; experience however shows that a calf may suffer under sudden conditions of restraint from what is conventionally expressed as 'nerves,' and therefore not only is this induction to a strange environment desirable but kindly treatment by all concerned is essential.[38]

After the operation, the abdomen was again covered with a dry apron, a wooden or bamboo collar was put around the calf's neck to keep it from licking the scratches, and it was put into a stall until the vesicles became ripe about five or six days later. The vesicles were harvested by scraping. The calf was again tied down to the table, the vesicles were soaked in warm water, and a few brushes with a cloth would remove as much of the crust as possible. After another wash, a Volkman's spoon would be used to scrape each row of vesicles with a single sweep to avoid mixing blood with the lymph. If the depot used the seed lymph in fresh rather than preserved form, harvesting involved conducting the scraping operation on the "stock vaccine" calf in the centre of the operation room, surrounded by "paste calves". After gathering vesicles from the former, the vesicles would be pricked to allow the lymph to ooze out onto spatulas which would be used to inoculate the paste calves. One vaccine stock calf was needed for every five paste calves.[39]

These procedures generally remained the same until the 1930s, when the vaccine depot in Meiktila adopted the "Malayan" method of cow vaccination. In 1934, the depot's director, G. H. Blaker, went to Kuala Lumpur (British Malaya) to study this method as it yielded a greater quantity of lymph than other methods. It involved washing the cow and then slaughtering it, allowing more lymph to be extracted from the animal. This method was adopted in Meiktila as the standard procedure by 1938 with one modification. Rather

[38] King, *Vaccination in the Tropics*, 31.

[39] Entrican, *Notes for the Use of Vaccinators*, 29–30; King, *Vaccination in the Tropics*, 4, 30, 33.

than wash the animal before slaughter, as in Kuala Lumpur, the animal was washed after slaughter in Meiktila. The adoption of this method reduced expenditure at the depot, as now fewer cattle had to be vaccinated, which meant fewer had to be bought.[40]

A regular supply of potable water was necessary for keeping the animals, the buildings, and the staff clean, for removal of sewage, and for drinking. On occasion, it was necessary to pour water over the calf sheds to bring down the temperatures inside. One of the considerations that led to the shift from Taunggyi was that Meiktila had greater access to fresh water, mainly from a large lake in the centre of town. The problem which remained, however, was how to harness this water for the depot's use. King had suggested in the 1920s that it should be possible to distribute water to a depot by means of gravity, and that it would be ideal if the water had "sufficient fall" so that it could be harnessed to generate electricity. However, Meiktila was built on a flat plain and this was not possible. From the 1910s, directors of the depot became very vocal about the need to improve the water supply. But mechanical aid was not forthcoming until 1927, when an electric pump was installed, which made it possible to draw water from the lake to fill the reservoirs at the depot. This was followed by an improved system of water supply in 1930, and, in 1933, the depot added a second Roturbo pump to one already in operation.[41]

Generally, the buildings and organisation of the depot evolved in tandem with growing concerns over cattle hygiene at every stage of the cultivation and harvesting process, and also as a result of the depot's growing output, which required more space, a larger staff, and a greater specialisation of tasks. When the Taunggyi vaccine depot was built in 1896, it was a mud and mat-walled building, which contributed, it was believed, to mouldy lymph, in the civil dispensary compound. This single building was divided into three rooms, the first, with an operating table for inoculation and harvesting the lymph, the second for post-operative stabling, and the third to store

40 *Report on the Administration of Burma for the Year 1933–34*, 117 [hereafter *RAB* followed by the year]; *Report on the State of Public Health in Burma during 1938*, 64.

41 King, *Vaccination in the Tropics*, 25; *NSVB for 1909–10*, 3; *NSVB for 1911–1912*, 4; *Annual Report of the Public Health Commissioner with the Government of India for 1927*, 141 [hereafter *RPHC* followed by the year]; *NSVB for 1929–30*, 9; *RAB for 1932–33*, 96.

equipment and fodder as well as prepare the vaccine paste. The last director of the Taunggyi vaccine depot recorded in his reports his frustration with the poor equipment he was allowed. It consisted only of the minimum necessary to prepare vaccine paste, including glass pestles, mortars, watch-glasses, bottles, a scraper, and a scale. Working conditions in the Meiktila depot were slightly better because the government allocated 1,100 rupees for the purchase of the land and apparatus. When it was opened in 1902, however, the depot consisted of only a single rented bungalow, with, one must assume, only space for basic functions. In addition, the depot suffered from poor management, which drew criticism from the superiors in Rangoon who carried out early inspections.[42]

Unlike Taunggyi, Meiktila was eventually given increased funding in the form of a special imperial government grant of 50,000 rupees in 1913 for expanding the number and size of its buildings. This resulted in the opening of a new laboratory and other buildings on 1 April 1915. To make a case for funding, the director of the depot, Williams, coincidentally the same person who had served as the director of the vaccine depot at Taunggyi a decade or so earlier, argued that expansion was necessary because of the depot's increased workload. Since Meiktila's production of lymph had gone up by 300 per cent, compared to 1903–1904, this was a difficult argument to ignore. However, there was more to the new buildings than just more space. They were built at a time of growing institutional awareness about the kind of buildings best suited for vaccine depots. It was now realised, for example, that "specially designed buildings" could help offset varying temperatures, which could rise substantially during the course of a day, or across seasons. A demand of successive directors in Meiktila was that stabling for calves be increased. This reflected a concern shared by other depots in British India, which recognised the need to house animals at each critical stage of cultivation and harvesting in separate buildings. King recommended, on the basis of his experiences in both Burma and Madras, that a vaccine institute should have separated waiting sheds where animals could be accommodated between the

42 "Annual Report on the Working of the Taunggyi Vaccine Depot for 1899–1900", xiii, xv; IOR/P/6034 File No. 1Z-5, Government Order, Rangoon, dated 31 May 1901; *TRVB for 1899–1900 to 1901–1902*, 5; *NSVB for 1899–1900*, 15, 16; *NSVB for 1902–03*, 3.

quarantine and inoculation periods; buildings for cleaning, shaving, and disinfecting animals; and buildings for the observation and treatment of questionable cases. He went on to say there should be inoculation sheds, which would include separate sections for vaccine stock and paste animals; an operation room; a vaccine preparation room; a cold storage; rooms for administration and storage; rooms for storing the clothes of those on duty, and for sterilising human clothing, and the cloth used on the animals; rooms for inoculation and care of calves; and rooms for staff accommodation. Besides, there would have to be buildings to provide power for ventilation and refrigeration, and to generate light and heat.[43]

What King recommended was an ideal situation, but Meiktila eventually adopted many of these arrangements, though with substantial delays compared to its counterparts on the subcontinent. The last major burst of construction at the depot, in 1930–31, brought about a number of improvements. For the first time, in 1931, Meiktila was equipped with a post-scraping stable. Though passing the vaccine lymph through cycles, including rabbits and guinea pigs, had become regular in Meiktila in the 1910s, a rabbit and guinea pig house, separate from the other buildings was not built until 1930, and water supply for this building was organised only a year later. A special quarters for the director was also added to the depot. Other construction during this period included improvements to old buildings. Equipment was also updated with the addition of a new operation theatre and a new operating table.[44]

## *Cattle Health*

The depot's dependence on cattle and other animals made animal health one of its significant concerns. Officers such as King believed that vaccination would not make an animal's health deteriorate in a well-run vaccine institute. In reality, what happened was that the animal's health showed a definite improvement because of the hygienic care and wholesome food it received. Diet was seen

43 *NSVB for 1911–12*, 4; *NSVB for 1912–13*, 4; *NSVB for 1914–15*, 4; *NSVB for 1915–16*, 4; King, *Vaccination in the Tropics*, 24, 27.

44 *RAB for 1929–30*, 102; *RAB for 1930–31*, 83; *RAB for 1931–32*, 139; *RAB for 1932–33*, 96.

as having an important effect on vesicle production, and for this reason, the depot had to ensure that it had access to fresh fodder throughout the year. Since the Meiktila depot did not have the support of the Civil Veterinary Department until the 1920s, the staff was very much on its own while tackling animal diseases and maintaining its cattle in good health. The depot also functioned as an unofficial cattle hospital. The British civil surgeons, indigenous clerks, and an "attendant", whose job was vaccinating calves and collecting and distributing animal lymph, also had to segregate and quarantine calves during outbreaks of epizootics. There were also indigenous "menial" workers who handled the day-to-day cleaning and feeding of the calves.[45]

It was especially important to look out for signs of disease, for once an animal disease was introduced to the depot, "its eradication may become a difficult matter". Epizootics such as rinderpest, anthrax, foot-and-mouth disease (*aftosa* or aphthouse fever), and hæmorrhagic septicæmia (*Pasteurella Multocida*) frequently devastated Burma's animal stocks before inoculations for rinderpest and anthrax were developed. When the animals were brought to the depot, they were subject to five days' quarantine, an interval that covered the incubation period of most cattle diseases. During this time, a quick inspection was conducted to determine that the calf did not have anthrax, fever, foot-and-mouth disease, or rinderpest. The initial indicators of good health to look for were soft and glossy hair free from parasites, a cool muzzle, and a fat and healthy looking body. Second, an examination of the mouth and hooves for sores was undertaken while the anus was examined for bloody discharge or diarrhoea, the nostrils for discharge, and the neck and stomach for swelling. If any doubts remained, a thermometer was resorted to. In the case of ticks, a quick spray with kerosene or smearing the hide with the raw mashed pulp of the weed *Leucas cephalotes* sufficed. Even after this quick inspection, the calf was observed for a week to make sure that it remained healthy. Only then was the animal vaccinated.[46]

45 King, *Vaccination in the Tropics*, 25–26; Entrican, *Notes for the Use of Vaccinators*, 28; "Annual Report on the Working of the Taunggyi Vaccine Depot for 1899–1900", xiv.

46 Entrican, *Notes for the Use of Vaccinators*, 28; King, *Vaccination in the Tropics*, 26, 28–29.

Despite these precautions, disease frequently found its way to the depot's herd, reducing the available number of healthy cattle. The outbreak of epidemics in the herd was feared because it could upset the lymph production process in many ways. Foot-and-mouth disease, rinderpest, anthrax, and haemorrhagic septicæmia claimed many cattle. Eighteen calves were stricken in an epidemic of foot-and-mouth disease and cow plague during 1902–03. In 1909, during the hot season, from March to May, the depot was hit by both foot and mouth and rinderpest, which killed 91 calves. At the end of the year, an outbreak of hæmorrhagic septicæmia increased the tally to 150, or about half the depot's cattle stock. The following year, 88 calves were killed by the same diseases,[47] seriously hindering the depot's production of vaccine. The director of the depot complained in 1909–10, "Much difficulty was experienced in maintaining the strain of vaccine lymph, owing to the prevalence of these epizootics and the difficulty experienced in obtaining healthy calves for operation".[48] Another difficult period came in 1925, after the Forest Department set up a camp in a forest reserve for the depot's grazing needs. A forest fire almost destroyed the camp, later, but the cattle stock was hit by a series of diseases from about the time it opened. The herd first suffered from foot-and-mouth disease, followed by rinderpest, and finally an outbreak of hæmorrhagic septicæmia, the last alone killing 59 calves.[49] In 1928, it was reported that an outbreak of rinderpest and foot-and-mouth disease caused "great anxiety and financial loss" to the department. This outbreak of epizootics was so severe that the Veterinary Department was requested to provide advice on how to prevent future outbreaks, and a plan and estimate for setting up a quarantine stable were quickly submitted to the government for sanction.[50] These infectious diseases killed many cattle, and weakened otherwise healthy animals, while the staff at the vaccine depot was often unable to maintain the efficacy of the strain of vaccine lymph operative at the time.

Different animal epidemics had differing effects on the depot's cattle stock. Rinderpest, "the most devastating bovine disease",

47 *TRVB for 1908–09 to 1910–11*, 6–7; *NSVB for 1909–1910*, 3.

48 *NSVB for 1909–10*, 3.

49 *TRVB for 1923–24 to 1925–26*, 10–11.

50 *NSVB for 1899–1900*, 11; *TRVB for 1899–1900 to 1901–1902*, 4–5; *TRVB for 1908–09 to 1910–11*, 7; *TRVB for 1926–27 to 1928–29*, 16.

was highly fatal but "bestow[ed] relatively solid immunity on survivors". It contaminated the equipment and stables for only a short period. So, though the stock was severely depleted, no major overhaul of facilities was required. Foot-and-mouth disease was an especially persistent and ubiquitous ailment that required dealing with the animal's environment as much as the aniınal itself, for it conferred a "permanent epidemic status" on affected areas if the disease was not eradicated. Depopulation of animal stock was only part of the solution, the animal's living area had to be disinfected, and the stables vacated for at least a month.[51] In several Burmese vaccine depots, such outbreaks necessitated a complete overhaul of the calf sheds at a time when space was required for quarantining the vulnerable cattle. Animal epidemic outbreaks were also costly because the vaccine depots had to continue feeding a large stock of calves without being able to dispose of them, in part because diseases such as the cow plague were spread mainly through cattle trading.[52]

Cooperation with the Veterinary Department was a late colonial development. The earliest significant intersection of Veterinary and Vaccination Department activities in Burma was in the late 1910s, when the Rangoon vaccine depot slaughtered its cattle after extracting the lymph so that the carcasses could be examined by a veterinary officer. The officer had to certify it free of disease if the lymph was to be issued for vaccination.[53] In the 1920s, however, lymph depots throughout British India were told by their superiors to cooperate more with the Veterinary Department to identify and prevent animal diseases. In Bombay, the depot staff was instructed

[51] Kahrs, *Viral Diseases of Cattle*, 278, 293, 299.

[52] *NSVB for 1899–1900*, 11; *NSVB for 1909–10*, 3; Kahrs, *Viral Diseases of Cattle*, 298.

[53] *TRVB for 1917–18 to 1919–20*, 4. This followed the prevailing method in Britain. The main concern was to avoid tuberculosis, though King recommended that in case of doubt, the tuberculin test could be resorted to and the Meiktila depot appears to have followed suit. There were two advantages in doing so. First, it was less costly, since the unnecessary elimination of expensive animals was avoided and, second, killing the calves would have been offensive to Hindus. This was also true of the Burmese Buddhists, who believed that the taking of life was a sin, although unlike the Hindus, they did not oppose the use of calves in cultivating vaccine. King, *Vaccination in the Tropics*, 26.

to work with the Veterinary Department to prevent outbreaks of rinderpest. The Lahore Institute (Punjab) turned to the Veterinary Department to set up their observation stables. The Patwa depot (United Provinces) even sent laboratory assistants to the Muktesar Imperial Laboratory for short courses on cattle disease. Elsewhere in British Asia, similar cooperation was in evidence. In the Federated Malay States, for example, veterinary officers inspected cattle before they were put on trains and sent to the vaccine depot in Kuala Lumpur. As for Burma, the Vaccination Department recommended that the depot communicate with staff of the Veterinary Department to keep track of the current status of animal diseases, and to detect animals at the depot that could be carrying foot-and-mouth disease. Identifying a case of foot-and-mouth disease had implications that went beyond the immediate concerns of the depot because the animal's entire history became the subject of a detailed and careful enquiry to ensure that resting places along the way and the railway cars used to transport it were properly disinfected.[54]

## *Conclusion*

The shift in the mode of transportation of vaccine lymph from arm-to-arm to cow-to-arm was not easy in Burma despite the lack of opposition based on religion as had initially occurred in other parts of British India. However, this change gradually gained ground with the establishment of a local vaccine depot to raise animal lymph. The local vaccine depot represented a turning point in the scope of the activities of the vaccination establishment in Burma by extending its fields of required knowledge. In the past, civil officers and vaccinators had operated through civil hospitals and dispensaries, conducting vaccination operations and reporting on their results. The challenge of establishing a local depot, however, required a journey into new areas of knowledge that went far beyond medical training. Determining the most suitable location for setting up a well-functioning vaccine depot required shifting attention to a number of new factors. Since the vaccine depot required access to healthy cattle throughout the year, the Vaccination Department's

[54] *RPHC for 1924*, 78–79; *Annual Report of the Medical Department (Federated Malay States) for 1931*, 195; King, *Vaccination in the Tropics*, 28–29.

first task was identifying a site at a relatively high altitude that had a suitable climate, access to water and good grazing grounds, proximity to the railways for the distribution of the vaccine lymph to various stations, markets for buying and selling calves, and a stable administration that could keep "dacoits" away. After the vaccine depot was opened, its staff had to develop an expertise in animal health, for acquiring, maintaining, and using cattle for the cultivation of lymph demanded that close attention be paid to the animals' diet, hygiene, and health.

With its expanded scope of operations and "fields of knowledge", the vaccination establishment in Burma found itself operating within a new "medical map" defined by the transportation infrastructure. For those administering vaccinations, formerly isolated civil stations connected only by river systems now became more accessible through a network of roads and the railways. All these areas came under the immediate supervision of the department. Places further out, away from the railway tracks, roads, and river banks, became more clearly defined as a shadowy hinterland, where operations would depend on the "unreliable" services of indigenous vaccinators.

As the vaccination establishment soon discovered, the opening of a vaccine depot at Taunggyi proved to be a short-lived solution to its problems. The limitations in the establishment's understanding of Burma's topography and climate contributed to the brevity of the Taunggyi depot's existence as also the changes that came about in the transportation infrastructure. The immediate result was the selection of a new site, Meiktila, for a new vaccine depot. What follows discusses how Meiktila was transformed into a laboratory to find the best preservative for lymph.

# 3

# *The Preservation of Lymph*

Changing approaches to lymph and vaccination helped to make research on lymph in Burma possible. Civil surgeons in the province were solving, at the local level, the problems they had in obtaining cows for vaccination purposes. Expanding vaccination operations in Burma coincided with the development of global scientific research into vaccine preservatives. New preservation methods, including glycerine, lanoline, vaseline, and chloroform, were of importance to the vaccine depot in Meiktila, as the province was in a tropical zone that deprived the lymph of its efficacy very fast. The development of a state railway system speeded up the transfer of lymph to a growing number of places, thus ushering in the right conditions for experiments in new methods of preserving lymph. The research in the Meiktila vaccine depot was hampered by poor funding and logistical challenges, but it was crucial to overcoming the problem of ineffective vaccine lymph, and demonstrating to the Burmese that vaccination was safe and effective. Here we examine the challenges faced by researchers in Meiktila and the successes they enjoyed.

## *Preserving Lymph*

In 1889, the vaccination establishment in Burma committed itself to preserved animal lymph, as opposed to direct vaccination from arm or calf. This change was a result of two developments, which were almost simultaneous. One was relevant only to Burma and the other to all the provinces in British India. First, the scale of vaccination operations from 1889 grew so much that the demand for lymph outstripped what civil surgeons and vaccinators in district stations could cultivate on their own. Although Upper Burma was annexed at the beginning of 1886, after the Third Anglo-Burmese War the previous year, the pacification campaign that followed continued for years. A systematic vaccination programme was introduced to Upper Burma only in 1889 when a scheme was initiated for "supplying the means of vaccination" to the new districts in the annexed territory. This included appointing vaccinators to all the districts in the province.[1] Even when vaccination work had been limited to Lower Burma, a delta with a better transportation infrastructure (by rivers and rail), district civil surgeons had found it necessary to rely on preserved lymph from Rangoon because it was difficult to obtain healthy calves, and parents were reluctant to allow their children to be taken to faraway villages. These problems were magnified in diffusely populated Upper Burma, where, in addition to active resistance to the British, transport facilities were inadequate, and civil surgeons found themselves far from reliable sources of vaccine lymph. In these circumstances, preserved lymph was a necessity.

The second development in 1889 was that the Government of India directed provincial governments to end arm-to-arm vaccination in favour of animal lymph, whether through direct calf-to-arm vaccination or through preserved lymph obtained by establishing animal lymph depots.[2] In the same year, Surgeon-Major Barclay submitted a report to Charles Haukes Todd Crosthwaite, the Chief Commissioner of British Burma (1887–90), recommending that these steps be taken. However, Crosthwaite was unwilling to act until "it was proved that the activity of the [animal] lymph could be maintained in this province for a considerable period".[3] His concern was based on his knowledge of local experiences with lymph, which, unless kept in the form of crusts, lost its vigour in a matter of hours.[4] As King, a prominent figure in the lymph preservation debate, first in Madras and then in Burma, observed, "It was . . . notorious that animal lymph could not be transported, and yet retain its vitality under tropical

[1] *RVB for 1889–90*, 1.

[2] IOR/P/7796, Burma File, 1908, Colonel W. G. King to Secretary to the Government of Burma, 10 January 1908, in Home (Medical) Department, Burma, January 1908, OIOC.

[3] *RVB for 1889–90*, 2.

[4] Ibid.

conditions".[5] Local governments now faced the task of finding a way to preserve lymph that would allow it to survive transport. As King explained, by 1890, there was very little information available on the preservation of lymph in India and local research seemed to be the answer.[6]

Though civil surgeons in Burma had complained for decades that stored lymph frequently failed in the tropical environment, they had not identified why it happened. Many civil surgeons complained in their reports that lymph lost its efficacy rapidly. O. E. Evans, the civil surgeon in Akyab, reported that locally raised lymph deteriorated within 48 hours, causing inflammation of the vesicles, which led to "ulcers and secondary abscesses".[7] Civil surgeons in Burma (and the subcontinent) had noticed the growth of extraneous organisms in the lymph that rapidly eroded its efficacy. Several decades of bacteriological research in Europe had preceded Evans's complaint. Between 1868 and 1886, researchers in Europe detected extraneous organisms in the lymph, but believed them to be the carriers or generators of smallpox. New research carried out between 1887 and 1891 found that these and other bacteria were not peculiar to the lymph, and could not have been contaminating it. Several years later, S. Monckton Copeman (1862–1947) demonstrated that the multiplication of bacteria was responsible for the opacity of lymph stored in capillary tubes, and for the deterioration in its vitality. But before they knew of this, doctors in Burma directed their attention to the effects of temperature. As a result, they found themselves unable to account for anomalies that seemed to run counter to the temperature theory. For instance, W. P. Kelly, the Superintendent for Vaccination in Burma, said in 1871 that he was confused why, on some occasions, lymph stored in hermetically sealed glass tubes deteriorated more rapidly when it was cool (85 degrees Fahrenheit, or 29 degrees Celsius, and below) than when it was hot (98 to 100 degrees Fahrenheit, or 36 to 38 degrees Celsius).[8]

[5] IOR/P/7796, Burma File, 1908, Colonel W. G. King to the Secretary to the Government of Burma, 10 January 1908, in Home (Medical) Department, Burma, January 1908, OIOC.

[6] Ibid.

[7] *RVB for 1889–90*, 5.

[8] *Report of the Medical Officer for 1895–96*, 283–285; *RVB for 1870–71*, 9.

The person mainly responsible for the distribution of preserved animal lymph in Burma from the early 1880s was Pedley, the Health Officer in Rangoon. Trials in the cultivation of animal lymph had been undertaken in 1883 in Thayetmyo, Toungoo, and Rangoon. They were most successful in Rangoon under Pedley's supervision and it was decided that the city would supply stations outside it with animal lymph crusts when calf-to-arm vaccinations using local calves proved difficult. Although there were occasional failures in the Rangoon vaccine depot, Pedley successfully carried out vaccinations in three consecutive years (1886 to 1889) using the calf-to-arm method, obviating the need for experiments with ways to preserve the lymph. Nevertheless, he sent significant numbers of lymph tubes to areas outside the municipality. Here, success or failure was usually attributed to the handling of the lymph by the vaccinator in question, not the quality of the lymph itself.[9]

## *Glycerine*

From 1889, Burma began to experiment with glycerine as a preservative for animal vaccine lymph. Barclay suggested that lymph could be protected from the high temperatures in the province by packing it in glauber's salts (sodium sulphate), but this idea made little headway.[10] Crosthwaite, however, did take Barclay's caution against the use of lymph kept in the form of crusts seriously, and ordered that experiments be undertaken "with regard to the possibility of effectually preserving lymph".[11] Pedley undertook experiments in December 1889 on ascertaining the effect of Burma's climate on stored lymph by investigating the relationship between the duration a specimen was stored and its effectiveness. Since he was looking at the effect of temperature, there was no single control group of vaccine lymph. On various days in the cold and hot seasons, Pedley scraped sixth-day vesicles from a calf, mixed them with glycerine (glycerol), and used them to vaccinate

9 *RVB for 1889–90*, 5.

10 IOR/P/7796, Burma File, 1908, Colonel W. G. King to the Secretary to the Government of Burma, 10 January, 1908, in Home (Medical) Department, Burma, January 1908, OIOC.

11 *RVB for 1889–90*, 2.

groups of prisoners, ranging from 10 to 170, in the Rangoon Central Jail.[12] An examination of his published experimental data indicates that some batches of glycerinated lymph produced progressively better results over the course of being stored one, two, three, and four or more weeks in the cold season. Meanwhile, batches of glycerinated lymph collected in the hot season improved slightly or retained the same level of vitality for only about a week before declining on a daily basis. Since different batches of lymph were used, there were anomalies that could be attributed to the proper or improper preparation of one batch or another. The general findings, summarised in the report on vaccination for that year, said,

> Different specimens of lymph paste collected and prepared in the cool months give very different results independent altogether of the interval that elapses between the collection of the lymph and the operation.[13]

Nevertheless, it was noted that glycerinated lymph stored for longer periods often gave much better results than lymph recently collected. Pedley, however, advised that given the unpredictability of lymph stored in this way, and the fact that it was more effective if used within 24 hours of collection, it should be used quickly in Rangoon. But for the storage of lymph that had to be transported outside Rangoon, glycerine was an improvement. Shortly after Pedley's 1889–90 trials, glycerine became freely used in Burma, for Rangoon was now able to produce glycerinated calf lymph that remained reasonably active long enough for distribution throughout the province.[14]

Pedley was unaware that the phenomenon he mistook for unpredictability would soon become one of the most important discoveries on preserving lymph. The glycerine was why the stored lymph improved over time. Glycerine was first identified by Michael-Eugène Chevreul (1786–1889) who, from 1811, had borrowed the methods of making soap to understand the basic principles of mutton fat. Heating mutton fat with caustic soda and purifying the residue, he extracted a clear, sweet-tasting liquid, which he named glycerine after the Greek word for "sweet".[15] It

12 *RVB for 1889–90*, 5.

13 Ibid., 6.

14 *RVB for 1889–90*, 5–6; *TRVB for 1890–91 to 1892–93*, 9.

15 Caroline M. Pond, *The Fats of Life* (Cambridge: Cambridge University Press, 1998), 7.

took nearly three decades after he published his findings in 1823 for glycerine to be added to both human and animal lymph to augment its quantity without reducing its effectiveness. In 1850, R. R. Cheyne had found that adding glycerine to human vaccine lymph was a better method than keeping lymph dried on points, believing that this was because the glycerine merely delayed decomposition. By 1869, research in Europe established that the properties of vaccine lymph remained unimpaired when one part of it was diluted with three parts of glycerine. Until the late 1880s, glycerine was thus viewed mainly as a handy diluent to increase the volume of vaccine lymph available for vaccination, or, as Cheyne showed, as a preservative. The experiments of O. Leoni and Pedley, both in 1889, also uncovered the germicidal effect of glycerine on micro-organisms in the vaccine lymph. However, Leoni's findings were not published until 1894, and Pedley failed to connect the improvement in the lymph with the glycerine he had used. Further, Pedley, for unclear reasons, resigned as Health Officer of Rangoon on 16 June 1890, bringing his experiments with glycerinated lymph to an end. So, when Copeman revealed the results of his experiments in a paper delivered at the International Congress of Hygiene in London in 1891, his discovery was the first to enter the general discourse on the relationship between glycerine and the preparation of lymph. He related how he had stored, in sealed capillary tubes, an emulsion of one part vesicle pulp mixed with two parts of .50 per cent pure glycerine in distilled water solution and found that extraneous organisms progressively declined over the course of several weeks. In 1896, researchers in Berlin found that the addition of glycerine with distilled water at 15 to 20 times the weight of the vesicle pulp did not reduce the effectiveness of the lymph. As glycerine promised to both purify and augment the supply of vaccine lymph, its use spread throughout continental Europe. In Britain, after the promulgation of the Vaccination Act of 1898, the National Vaccine Establishment began distributing glycerinated calf lymph on 1 January 1899.[16]

[16] *Report of the Medical Officer for 1895–96*, xxviii, 283, 285, 286, 287, 288; Kinyoun, "The Action of Glycerin on Bacteria in the Presence of Cell Exudates", 725; MacNalty and Craig, "Sydney Arthur Monckton Copeman, 1862–1947", 40–42.

## *Lanoline*

Despite the seemingly complete victory of glycerine, lanoline soon emerged as a serious competitor, at least in British India.[17] In Madras, King conducted experiments with lanoline. Lanoline (sometimes known at the time as wool grease) is a greasy, water-repellent secretion produced by wool-bearing animals, such as sheep. King found that by reducing vaccine vesicles to a pulp and mixing it with lanoline into a paste, he could sustain the efficacy of the lymph for 40 days. This period was likely to be prolonged if purified lanoline was used. King's findings, which made a strong case for the use of lanoline, drew the favourable attention of the Government of India. Glycerinated lymph was quite resistant to contamination and was easy to operate with. However, it did not last longer than 10 to 14 days in high temperatures. Lanolinated lymph had a longer life span than glycerinated lymph, from about three weeks to a month. However, it was more difficult to handle, making it more susceptible to contamination.[18]

The lanoline method was brought to Burma by an unusual series of events. King's success with lanoline in Madras was interrupted in 1892 when he was removed from the post of deputy sanitary commissioner for having distributed calf lymph without the government's permission. The British government eventually pressured the Madras government to revoke his removal in September 1893, promoting him to sanitary commissioner for Madras.[19] In the interim, however, he found a temporary post in Mandalay and used the opportunity to demonstrate his method of preparing lanolinated lymph to the civil surgeons posted to Burma. When the doctors returned to their stations and tried lanoline on their own, however, the results varied. In Akyab and Maulmain, for example, lanoline paste from Bangalore had a success rate of 76.6 per cent to 86.5 per cent, while in Monywa, it had a lower percentage of success than fresh lymph. Surgeon-Captain Basu,

17 Bhattacharya, Harrison, and Worboys, *Fractured States*, 194–95.

18 IOR/P/7796, Burma File, 1908, Colonel W. G. King to the Secretary to the Government of Burma, 10 January, 1908, in Home (Medical) Department, Burma, January 1908, OIOC; *RVB for 1891–92*, 8; *TRVB for 1902–03 to 1904–05*, 4.

19 These events are related in Harrison, *Public Health in British India*, 86.

the civil surgeon in Minbu, found that lanoline paste also caused glandular inflammations and the eruption of boils. King dismissed such problems, attributing them to civil surgeons not strictly following his preparation methods. At his insistence, the commissioner in Mandalay dispatched officers to the Bangalore institute where they were properly trained in King's methods of cultivating lymph and preserving it with lanoline. The officers circulated these methods throughout the province on their return.[20] However, King was of the opinion that the cultivation and preservation of lymph by local surgeons was not up to the mark. He argued that the production of lymph in small and isolated depots scattered around the province could not be trusted, and if lanolinated lymph was to be properly prepared, it had to be done at a "single, well-organised vaccine institute", which could produce sufficient lymph to meet both ordinary demand and that during epidemics. Commenting in 1892, however, P. W. Dalzell, the officiating Sanitary Commissioner for Burma, desired more proof of the superiority of lanoline's preservative qualities before any such move was made.[21]

## *Vaseline*

Glycerine and lanoline were not the only preservatives tried out in British India. In 1895, Major Charles James Bamber of the IMS began research in Multan in Punjab using vaseline (petroleum jelly). Punjab was a different case to Madras and Burma. There, indigenous resistance to the use of bovine lymph was very strong, leading the vaccination establishment to abandon its use and rely solely on buffalo lymph. As buffalo calves did not yield enough lymph, it was decided to build up a supply over time, thus making it necessary to preserve the lymph. King's work had raised the possibility that alternatives to glycerine might be better for the Indian climate. Since his work had underlined the weaknesses of glycerine in the tropical context, Bamber turned to vaseline.

20 *TRVB for 1890–91 to 1892–93*, 9; *RVB for 1891–92*, 8; IOR/P/7796, Burma File, 1908, Colonel W. G. King to the Secretary to the Government of Burma, 10 January 1908, in Home (Medical) Department, Burma, January 1908, OIOC.

21 *RVB for 1891–92*, 8.

Vaseline had been invented in 1859 but had only become widely available in the 1870s when it was promoted as a healing agent. It was used to preserve lymph in Europe, particularly Germany, as mentioned in an 1890 report by M. Bauer. While King's favoured lanoline was an animal product, vaseline was not, making its use in preserving lymph more acceptable to the Hindus in Punjab.[22]

Bamber began a comparative trial that tested white vaseline against samples of glycerine, lanoline paste he had prepared, and lanoline he had requested from Mysore. Glycerine performed the worst, becoming mouldy after only two weeks. While both the lanoline pastes did better than the glycerinated lymph, white vaseline yielded the best results. It also had a number of advantages over lanoline paste. Vaseline was easier to work with because it was more fluid and "less tenacious" than lanoline. While lanoline was opaque, medicinal vaseline was clear, making it easier to determine whether it had mixed correctly with the vesicles. Since vaseline was not organic, it was not prone to moulds, whereas this was a significant problem with lanoline and glycerine. Though another vaseline trial failed the following year, in 1896, this was blamed on poor preparation.[23] Vaseline lymph, it was argued, was a "putrescible substance and unless all instruments introduced into the tube are properly sterilised each time, decomposition is readily set up, and the lymph becomes bad". Another criticism of the vaseline vaccine was that it did not produce a "pitted appearance" on the vaccinated arm, which, as a rule, was taken as the sign of a successful vaccination.[24] In any case, it was concluded in 1896 that vaseline lymph performed just as well as the buffalo-to-arm method. Vaseline would remain the sole preservative of lymph in Punjab until W. F. Harvey of the IMS conducted new experiments in 1902 and 1903 comparing it with glycerine. He found glycerinated lymph superior, for it was easier than vaseline to mix with vaccine pulp, it yielded the characteristic

[22] Collier, "The Preservation of Vaccinia Virus", 79; *Report of the Medical Officer for 1895–96*, 291; *Report on Sanitary Measures in India for 1895–96*, 23, 100, 186; *Report on Sanitary Measures in India for 1899–1900*, 126, 229; Bhattacharya, Harrison, and Worboys. *Fractured States*, 48–49.

[23] *Report of the Medical Officer for 1895–96*, 291; *Report on Sanitary Measures in India for 1895–96*, 23, 100, 186; *Report on Sanitary Measures in India for 1899–1900*, 126, 229.

[24] *Report on Sanitary Measures in India for 1896–97*, 126.

scab, did not cause inflammation and pus as did vaselinated lymph, and could withstand higher temperatures.[25]

As civil surgeons in Burma continued their own trials of lanoline, glycerine and other preservatives for lymph, their superiors in the colonial medical establishment found themselves perplexed by the variety of opinions and experiences.

> These reports are so conflicting that at present no definite conclusions can be drawn as to the relative merits of the various preparations. Not only do the opinions of the Medical Officers differ widely regarding the best method of cultivation, and to storage of animal lymph but the results obtained by individual officers at different times with the same preparation have been very variable.[26]

Although, as we shall see, the Meiktila vaccine depot (later formally named the Burma Central Vaccine Depot) would make use of both lanoline and glycerine (eventually favouring the latter) for years, the Rangoon vaccine depot continued to produce only glycerinated lymph for the remainder of the colonial period, finding glycerine a satisfactory preservative in normal situations.[27] One contributing factor was that in 1895 and 1896, King's and Bamber's findings were rejected by F. R. Blaxall and Copeman in Britain, who criticised them for not having provided any "bacteriological evidence" on the germicidal value of lanoline or vaseline. Instead, it was asserted, these two agents had "little if any value" in preventing the growth of extraneous organisms during storage. Likewise, King's and Bamber's assertions that glycerinated lymph became mouldy very quickly were dismissed as evidence that the glycerinated lymph was "not properly prepared" or was "left exposed to the air". King and many other civil surgeons in the IMS were not persuaded by Copeman's views, and the question of whether glycerine or lanoline was best suited for the preservation of vaccine lymph in British India would be contested for the next few decades.[28]

25 *Report on Sanitary Measures in India for 1902–03*, 94; See Harvey's comments from 1912 on these findings in W. F. Harvey, "Vaccine Lymph Production, Preparation, and Preservation", *Indian Journal of Medical Research* 8 (1920–21), 262.

26 *RVB in Burma for 1891–92,* 8.

27 *NSVB for 1899–1900*, 14.

28 *Report of the Medical Officer for 1895–96*, xxviii–xxix, 291; Bhattacharya, Harrison, and Worboys, *Fractured States*, 181–88.

## *Research in Meiktila*

When the Vaccination Department in Burma established a central vaccine depot, first in Taunggyi and then in Meiktila, it merely hoped that the institution would soon be capable of meeting the demand for vaccine lymph from all over the province, except Rangoon. At first, there was no government mandate to carry out extensive experiments and even if there had been, Taunggyi was poorly equipped to do so. Even when the Meiktila vaccine depot was established in 1902, few new investigations into the preservation of lymph appear to have taken place. The first year of operation was a disaster. This appears to have been partly the result of the nature of official duties that the health officer had to perform. In the mid-nineteenth century, IMS doctors attached to Indian Army battalions stationed in the districts were seconded to the local civil stations and expected to carry out, in addition to their responsibilities in the cantonments, sanitary and medical work in the towns. For the rest of the century, the post frequently remained a collateral charge, its occupant being responsible for the administration of the local jail as well. When the Meiktila depot opened, its initial directors had all these responsibilities in addition to running what was meant to be a fully functioning vaccine production centre. That all this was too much for one officer to handle was brought to the notice of the government when the Inspector-General of Jails pointed out that this arrangement adversely affected the administration of local jails. Further, when this officer's tenure ended, no replacement could be found because the number of military assistant surgeons in the colony was considerably lower than needed. So, in 1903, the Government of Burma requested that the Government of India relieve the military surgeon in Meiktila of the collateral charge by appointing a full-time, second-class civil surgeon. The Government of India did so, in part because running the local jail required a permanent rather than temporary officer. Running the jail efficiently required fluency in both Burmese and "Hindustani" so that the appointee could get acquainted with the prisoners and become familiar with the institution's daily routine. However, the Government of India also expressed its recognition of what running the vaccine depot entailed.

> The establishment of a vaccine depot at Meiktila adds to the necessity for the appointment of a whole-time Civil Surgeon to that station. The work in connection with the depot, especially in its initiative stage, calls for close supervision and it is essential that the officer entrusted with the duty of obtaining calves, the cultivation of lymph, etc., should be a permanent resident of the station, otherwise the influence required to bring matters to a successful issue in obtaining material for the cultivation and propagation of good lymph, and for its regular and prompt distribution cannot be assured.[29]

Despite this change, much of the administration, for a variety of reasons, ranging from ill health to the exigencies created by World War I, remained temporary. Between 1902 and early 1904, the Meiktila depot was managed by three directors, Captain Penny, Lieutenant D. J. F. Donoghue, and Major T. W. Stewart. Over the course of the next 15 years, it would have 13 more directors. Nevertheless, the creation of the post of civil surgeon in Meiktila held out the hope of a more or less permanent appointment and one incumbent, Surgeon Major (and later Lieutenant-Colonel) Entrican (1865–1935) managed the depot at two different times (April 1904 to December 1908, and November 1917 to December 1919) for a total of six and a half years.[30] Entrican's role in the transformation of Meiktila into a research centre for vaccination in Burma lay in the numerous experiments he conducted. Such experiments depended on the individual in charge, since they changed rapidly (see Table 1). From late 1908, when Entrican left Meiktila, until he returned in November 1917, research at the depot noticeably declined.

The return of King to Burma in 1905, when he was appointed Superintendent General of Vaccination in Burma (1905–06) and then Sanitary Commissioner of Burma (1906–08), was fortuitous for Entrican. King, as we have seen, was an advocate of taking the tropical context into account and challenging the strongly held views on the superiority of glycerine in preparing and storing vaccine lymph. Research on the subject in Burma had been at a standstill

29 IOR/L/PJ/6/640 File 1413, J. B. Wingate to the Secretary to the Government of India, Home Department, 27 February 1903, Judicial and Public Papers (1903), OIOC.

30 *TRVB for 1902–03 to 1904–05,* 4; *NSVB for 1902–03*, 2; *NSVB for 1908–09*, 4; *NSVB for 1917–18*, 4; *RAB for 1919–20*, 167.

TABLE 1: Directors of the Meiktila Vaccine Depot, 1902–34

| *From* | *Until* | *Name* |
|---|---|---|
| 1 February 1902 | 8 March 1903 | Capt. Penny |
| 8 March 1903 | 2 April 1903 | Lt. D. J. F. O'Donoghue |
| 2 April 1903 | April 1904 | Maj. T. W. Stewart |
| April 1904 | December 1908 | Maj. J. Entrican |
| December 1908 | 1 April 1909 (temporary) | Capt. J. Good |
| 1 April 1909 | 26 November 1909 (official) | |
| 26 November 1909 | 26 February 1910 | Capt. E. A. Walker |
| 26 February 1910 | 23 March 1910 | Capt. R. D. Saigol |
| 23 March 1910 | 20 January 1912 | Capt. H. A. Dougan |
| 30 January 1912 | April 1912 | Maj. Dick |
| April 1912 | April 1913 | Maj. Beit |
| 1912–13 | | Capt. Munro (temporary)<br>Capt. Churchill (temporary)<br>Capt. Farebrother (temporary) |
| April 1913 | 16 September 1914 | Maj. E. A. Walker |
| 16 September 1914 | 1914 (late in year) | Lt. Col. Penny |
| 1914 (late in year) | March 1916 | Capt. L. K. Rodriguez |
| March 1916 | 26 November 1917 | Dr W. D. Jones |
| 26 November 1917 | December 1919 | Lt. Col. J. Entrican |
| December 1919 | 24 June 1920 | Capt. A. J. Symes |
| 24 June 1920 | 14 June 1923 | Capt. Aung Tun |
| 14 June 1923 | 19 February 1924 | Lt.-Col. H. A. Williams |
| 19 February 1924 | c. 1926 | Maj. J. W. Jones |
| c. 1926 | 1 March 1927 | H. H. Lynsdale |
| 1 March 1927 | June 1934 at the earliest, date unavailable | G. H. Blaker |

since Pedley's resignation almost 15 years earlier. King, who placed so much value on local research in India that his work in Madras was recognised by naming the new laboratories in Guindy the King Institute of Preventative Medicine in 1903, was eager to rekindle research in Burma. He immediately gave Entrican a mandate to turn the Meiktila vaccine depot into a virtual research facility and conduct experiments with the various lymph preservatives available. Finding the best preservation method to make the best use of locally cultivated vaccine lymph in a province that lacked proper transport facilities, was a serious challenge.[31]

During 1905–06, Entrican began comparative tests on lanolinated vaccine, glycerinated vaccine and quinated vaccine. While the virtues and drawbacks of glycerine and lanoline in the Indian subcontinent were well known in Burma, the properties of quinine and its possible preservative effect on lymph had yet to be examined. Some work had been done by Alan B. Green, a doctor in Britain, on the use of quinine as a germicidal agent to get rid of extraneous organisms. However, due to quinine's tendency to slowly modify the vesicle, he set aside these experiments. Entrican, as King pointed out at the time, was unfamiliar with this research. In his own work, Entrican developed a preservative of bihydrochloride of quinine in sterile mucilage and stained the mixture with cochineal. After a series of experiments, he successfully produced a vaccine that contained fewer micro-organisms. Entrican concluded that lanoline was preferable if "duration and vitality" were the priority. But considering that indigenous vaccinators in the colony were still not very skilful, he suggested that the more easily handled glycerine might be better for Burma until such time as the Burmese vaccinators became capable of handling lanoline. He would later attempt to achieve this through the establishment of the Meiktila Training School for Vaccination, of which more comes later. Entrican's concerns mirrored those of King, who had also advocated training indigenous vaccinators in careful procedures if lanoline were to be used. King lost no time in publicly endorsing Entrican's experiments and his conclusions.[32]

31 *TRVB for 1902–03 to 1904–05*, 4; *Times*, 5 April 1935, 18.

32 *TRVB for 1902–03 to 1904–05*, 4; *NSVB for 1905–06*, 3; *NSVB for 1906–07*, 3.

## *Entrican and Chloroform*

Entrican turned his attention to chloroform as a possible agent for rooting out extraneous organisms from the lymph before it was stored. The cleansing effect of chloroforming lymph had been established elsewhere. In 1906, Entrican reinvestigated the matter. The usual practice was to insert the preserved lymph into a glass receptacle, such as a capillary tube, and seal it with heat to help prevent more extraneous organisms from entering it during storage. Entrican attempted to improve upon this by filtering chloroform into the lymph, pushing chloroform-impregnated air through it, and using a current of air to carry away the excess chloroform. However, the experiment was deemed a failure when it was found that the efficacy of the chloroformed lymph did not exceed one week. It was presumed to be unsuitable for general use in Burma where lymph had to retain vitality for up to 20 days or more. Entrican also initially believed that chloroform was too expensive, "purchased out of all proportions to the advantage gained", and rejected using it on a daily basis. He then devised another method, dissolving bottling wax in a small amount of chloroform and adding it the moment the glycerinated lymph was sealed in the receptacle. Comparing the chloroformed specimens with a control group stored in the usual way, he found the chloroformed lymph was more effective in eliminating extraneous organisms. Moreover, while the normal method of chloroforming affected the vitality of the lymph, his new method did not. Entrican recommended, on the basis of his experiments and the results of field tests where lymph sealed in the new way did well in primary vaccinations, that these experiments be continued on a larger scale, a view supported by Williams, the Superintendent of Vaccination.[33] Subsequent trials in Burma revealed that chloroform did indeed affect lymph longevity, its use creating a situation in which "the cure is worse than the disorder". It was therefore abandoned in favour of experiments using vapour of amyl alcohol. Though these were more successful, the results were too marginal to suggest any change to the purification method. Meiktila abandoned attempts to use chloroform, but the process was picked up by vaccine institutes in India and used with some measure of success. Its use became routine in Belgaum (Bombay)

[33] *TRVB for 1905–06 to 1907–08*, 7; *NSVB for 1906–07*, 3.

from 1927, in Punjab (after successful trials from 1930) from 1933, and in the United Provinces from 1934, where it was used to treat especially bad lymph.[34]

## *Entrican and Filling Tubes*

Entrican's research on filling and sealing tubes continued but his main innovations had to do with increasing the speed and accuracy with which tubes were filled. A little "vaccine expeller" made of vulcanised rubber had been introduced in the Rangoon vaccine depot in 1900. Before that, the vaccinator had to put his lips to the tube and, through suction, draw the lymph out. With the "vaccine expeller", the lymph could be easily pushed out of the tube by the vaccinator. In reverse, glycerinated lymph could be drawn into the tube, allowing an assistant to fill, "accurately and rapidly", 80 to 100 tubes in 15 minutes. In 1906, Entrican produced two machines, about which, unfortunately, few technical descriptions are available. We do know that one filled tubes with lanoline vaccine and the other filled capillary tubes with glycerinated and quinated lymph. King praised each as "decidedly ingeniously contrived apparatus". They reduced several hours of "tedious" work to something that required only a few minutes. Vaccine depots on the subcontinent, beginning with those in Shillong (Assam), Lucknow, and Patwa Dangar (both in the United Provinces) in 1907, used replicas of Entrican's machines (crediting him for the inventions), observing that they had "revolutionised the laborious task of tube filling".[35]

In 1909, Entrican began attempts to modify the practice of sealing tubes by using heat. He tried using paraffin and wax, but the heat-sealing method was found to be 3.5 per cent more successful.[36] When he returned to Meiktila for his second stint as director, at a time when the depot issued only glycerinated lymph, Entrican was a strong advocate of continuing to rely on capillary tubes for distributing lymph. He argued that "no system that involves the

[34] *TRVB for 1917–18 to 1919–20*, 5; *RPHC for 1927*, 141; *RPHC for 1930*, 242; *RPHC for 1933*, 169; *RPHC for 1934*, 168; *RPHC for 1935*, 113.

[35] *NSVB for 1900–1901*, 3; *NSVB for 1905–06*, 3; *Report on Sanitary Measures in India for 1907–08*, 113, 115.

[36] *NSVB for 1909–10*, 3; *TRVB for 1908–09 to 1910–11*, 7.

use of bottles, collapsible leaden tubes, etc., each containing 20 to 50 doses, can approach the capillary tubes as a medium of distribution".[37] Nevertheless, for him, the best method of sealing the capillary tubes had yet to be found and he resumed experiments to find a better alternative to the heating method. First, the ends of the capillary tubes were plugged with a high concentration of gum acacia and plaster of Paris. These ends were then dipped into a resinous mixture that was impervious to moisture or air. Entrican stressed that excluding air was essential, partly because it prevented contamination but mainly because it "secur[ed] maximum longevity for the lymph".[38]

## *Difficulties at the Depot*

Despite Entrican's many experiments in 1905 and 1906, a range of problems, personal, professional and logistical, made both research and normal functioning of the depot difficult. Given the early role played by Entrican in setting the depot's research agenda and the length of time he served there, the wealth of archival material on Meiktila is connected with him and his work. This material affords us an unusually detailed look at the kind of challenges faced by many of the early twentieth century directors of the vaccine depots in British India.

Work in the Meiktila vaccine depot was continually hampered by the inefficient procedures that governed obtaining medical supplies in British India, especially in Burma. To conduct bacteriological investigations on the purity of the lymph cultivated at the depot and to seal capillary tubes, Entrican needed special equipment not stocked by government (medical) stores. His initial indent for these supplies was made in June 1904, but the first items reached Meiktila nearly a year later (11 months), some did not arrive until July and August 1907, and some had not turned up even in September 1907. A motor air engine indented for in May 1906 had not arrived 16 months later. When proper equipment was essential for carrying out experimental research and none of it was available locally,

37 *TRVB for 1917–18 to 1919–20*, 5.
38 Ibid.

waiting times of one year or more for supplies were "maddening", complained Entrican.[39]

With regard to medical supplies, the major handicap not mentioned by Entrican, but realised by others in government, was the status of Meiktila, which was originally intended to be only a vaccine depot. It was not a research institute, as many depots were officially becoming in other parts of British India. As a vaccine depot, Meiktila was subject to the rule that European manufactured goods had to be received from the Medical Stores Department or the Stores Department of India. In contrast, research institutes, including bacteriological and pathological laboratories, benefited from a permission granted by the Secretary of State of British India on 22 November 1901, which allowed them to buy the equipment and chemicals they needed directly from manufacturers or agents in Britain. Entrican's support of lanoline almost became moot because of new problems with the Medical Stores Department. It was not only slow, but also did not pay enough attention to the quality of the things it bought. In September 1906, a supply of lanoline indented for in May finally arrived and was put to immediate use. The depot's vaccine lymph was ruined and its work was very nearly brought to a halt by the time it was realised that this batch of lanoline was inferior. Lanoline brought in from Madras and Calcutta, both of which had presumably also acquired their supplies through the Medical Stores Department, was just as destructive. As the work of the depot was delayed by the lack of good lanoline for nearly six months, Entrican circumvented the rules and obtained a new and good supply from Burroughs and Wellcome in London. Not surprisingly, when he tried the lanoline he received from the Medical Stores Department again in May 1907, he found that it was just as bad as it had been the year before. Given these problems and their negative impact on the research activities in Meiktila, in 1908, the Indian government, at the request of the Government of Burma, sanctioned a special allowance to the Meiktila vaccine depot, which allowed it to buy its requirements directly. This marked the beginning of Meiktila's status as a quasi-research institute, now treated in reports in the same category as official research institutes in India such as the King

39 IOR/P/7786 Burma File 1908, Major J. Entrican to Superintendent of Vaccination, Burma, September 15, 1907, Home (Medical) Department, Burma, January 1908, OIOC.

Institute. A subsequent resolution by the Commerce and Industry Department the same year expanded the scope of this exemption, one now granted to the superintendents of all vaccine depots, by allowing it to purchase any item necessary for experiments or research from manufacturers or dealers not only in Britain, but also in the United States, Japan, or any other country where such items were made.[40]

The change in the equipment supply system helped ease potential problems in acquiring cooling technology. Burma's high temperatures had contributed to Meiktila's early failures in cultivating effective vaccine lymph.[41] During the hot season from April to June, the temperature rose to more than 100 degrees Fahrenheit, or 38 degrees Celsius, encouraging the growth of extraneous organisms. Until 1912, the Meiktila depot attempted to manufacture lymph during the cold season and rely on dry storage so that it could be used in the hot season. However, this limited the time for lymph cultivation, and prevented the accumulation of a stock large enough to meet provincial demand. Artificial refrigeration was the obvious solution, for keeping lymph at low temperatures had a good effect on it.

> Storage at a low temperature gradually reduces the extraneous organisms present in all lymph and since these are largely responsible for the violent and painful reaction that sometimes follows vaccination, their elimination is most desirable.[42]

In 1907, the Rangoon municipality sanctioned the construction of a new vaccine depot in the Kandawgalay ward, but it was not completed until the end of 1909. With state-of-the-art facilities, the Rangoon depot was able to begin experiments in early 1910 on the longevity of lymph kept in cold storage. The lymph was tested at intervals of three months and it revealed refrigeration was successful. Soon after, in Meiktila, Entrican's successor, Captain R. D. Saigol,

[40] Ibid; IOR/P/7786 Burma File 1908, D. Sherame to the Secretary to the Government of India, 23 January 1908; Colonel King to the Secretary to the Government of Burma, 8 October 1907, Home (Medical) Department, Burma, January 1908, OIOC; IOR/P/7786 Burma File 1908, P. W. Monie to the Secretary to the Government of Burma, 23 May 1908, Home (Medical) Department, Burma, January 1908, OIOC.

[41] *NSVB for 1903–04*, 3.

[42] *TRVB for 1917–18 to 1919–20*, 5.

tried out a cold storage box and thermos flasks to keep glycerinated lymph at a low temperature for just 10 days, but both failed to keep the lymph fresh. Although the Vaccination Department realised that what was really needed was a small refrigeration plant, it lacked the funds to buy such equipment. It took almost two years for the depot to be provided with sufficient funds to obtain powered refrigeration on a very limited scale, and a small, powered refrigerator was installed in 1912.[43]

Although refrigeration technology was regularly improved over the course of Meiktila's operations in the colonial period, it remained problematic. Poor funding also meant that when the cooling technology failed, it could take months or even years for approval to be granted for repairs or replacements. In 1914, two new cooling devices were installed. The first was a refrigeration plant powered by a natural gas and an oil engine. During 1915, this refrigerator ran well and allowed the Meiktila staff to preserve lymph for up to four months, representing a 1,200 per cent increase in longevity. Soon after, it began to break down frequently. Although the refrigerator itself began to work better in 1918, after it was completely overhauled, the natural gas and oil engines that powered it "caused endless trouble". Further, the fact that the engines and the refrigerator were housed in a building made of corrugated iron, meant excessive heat, and more difficulty in maintaining low temperatures. The second cooling device installed in 1914 was a small ice-making machine. This was powered by a gas engine, supplied by a gas generator and a gas tank, and could turn out 34 kilograms (75 pounds) of ice a day (an impressive capacity given the state of refrigeration technology at the time and the intense heat of the area). Attached to the ice machine was a chamber which could be used to store lymph, keeping it effective for at least 13 months. The ice machine operated successfully until 1929–30 when it was upgraded. The last major changes to cooling equipment in Meiktila during the colonial period were the addition of an ice-chest, similar to that used in the Dutch vaccine depot at Bandung, in 1927, which allowed the storage of lymph at temperatures below 10 degrees Celsius; and a Glacia G-10 ice

43 *NSVB for 1909–10*, 3, 4; *NSVB for 1911–12*, 4; *TRVB for 1908–09 to 1910–11*, 7; *NSVB for 1911–12*, 4.

plant in 1928, which was replaced by a larger Glacia G-20 ice plant in 1930.[44]

### *Lymph Production and Rejuvenation*

As Bhattacharya, Harrison, and Worboys point out, the declining use of lanolinated lymph in British India during the 1920s prompted research into other types of smallpox vaccine that would have greater efficacy in India's tropical environment such as rabbit neuro vaccine, dried lymph vaccine, and egg-culture-based vaccine. Such experiments failed and were abandoned by the end of the 1920s in favour of intensified efforts to improve the potency and purity of lymph, particularly seed lymph, which was believed to be one way to increase the yield and quality of bovine lymph. These efforts were in part motivated by the desire to solve the problems in acquiring a dependable supply of animals for lymph cultivation.[45]

Methods to test the potency of lymph had greatly improved since the nineteenth century, when potency could only be determined by observing the results it had on people who were vaccinated. This changed in 1901, when Albert Calmette and Jean Camille Guérin published a new method of testing potency using rabbits, which was improved by Guérin in 1905, allowing several dilutions of the virus. The test, which came to be known as the Calmette-Guérin international potency test, allowed for a much more accurate assessment of the potency of lymph and did away with some of the discomforts and dangers of human testing. Most vaccine institutes and depots in British India in the late 1920s and 1930s relied mainly on human testing, with the exception of the United Provinces, where rabbit testing was also done. Meiktila, however, adopted the Calmette-Guérin test, in conjunction with additional tests that were developed such as Cunningham's potency test for calves, until operations came to a halt during World War II. This was an important advantage because the greater accuracy of the

[44] *NSVB for 1915–16*, 4; *TRVB for 1917–18 to 1919–20*, 5, 8; *NSVB for 1914–15*, 4; *RAB for 1929–30*, 102; *TRVB for 1911–12 to 1913–14*, 8; *TRVB for 1914–15 to 1916–17*, 8; *RPHC for 1927*, 140–141; *RPHC for 1928*, 165; *NSVB for 1929–30*, 9.

[45] Bhattacharya, Harrison, and Worboys, *Fractured States*, 197.

Calmette-Guérin test made experiments in lymph preservation more meaningful.[46]

Entrican had begun research into maintaining the potency of the strain of vaccine during his first term as director of the Meiktila vaccine depot. He first attempted to improve the quality of the lymph by taking some of it from a child's vaccine vesicle and applying it to a scarification on a calf in a process known as retro-vaccination.[47] Retro-vaccination did not always work and its results were often poor. Though it would occasionally be used in tandem with other methods by some of Entrican's successors, such as Williams in 1912–13, it would never be the main method employed. Entrican then turned to the inoculation of rabbits to reinforce the strain of the virus, and this yielded better results. The number of rabbits through which the virus was passed changed (15 in 1906, 14 in 1914, 10 in 1915, and 21 in 1923) and, on a few occasions, it was passed through a buffalo calf and healthy children, but the method remained the same between 1906 and the early 1920s. One of the benefits of using rabbits as vaccinifers was that it saved the depot money, cattle being more expensive.[48] Another was that, by 1922, Burma had a vastly improved rate of success per operation (see Table 2).

Passing the virus through only one type of animal soon changed. Dutch doctor A. N. Nijland of the colonial Government Cowpox Establishment (first at Weltevreden, a suburb of Batavia, and then Bandung, in Java, from 1926) developed a method of purifying lymph and maintaining its potency that became widely known in British

46 *RPHC for 1928*, 165; *RPHC for 1929*, 165; *RPHC for 1930*, 242; *RPHC for 1932*, 194; *RPHC for 1933*, 169; *RPHC for 1934*, 168–69; *RPHC for 1935*, 113–14; *RPHC for 1936*, 181–82; *NSVB for 1929–30*, 10; *Report on the State of Public Health in Burma During 1939*, 60; Collier, "The Preservation of Vaccinia Virus", 76.

47 Bhattacharya, Harrison, and Worboys explain that retro-vaccination had begun early in the nineteenth century on the subcontinent. *Fractured States*, 38–39.

48 Entrican, *Notes for the Use of Vaccinators*, 28; *TRVB for 1905–05 to 1907–08*, 6; *TRVB for 1908–09 to 1910–11*, 7; *NSVB for 1912–13*, 4; *NSVB for 1914–15*, 4; *NSVB for 1915–16*, 4; *NSVB for 1923–24*, 7; the Belgaum Institute (Bombay) also kept up the potency of lymph by passing it through rabbits in 1924, 1929 and 1930. *RPHC for 1924*, 79; *RPHC for 1929*, 165; *RPHC for 1930*, 242.

TABLE 2: Vaccination Operations, 1901–31

| *Year* | *Success rate of primary vaccinations (per cent)* | *Success rate of revaccinations (per cent)* | *Total operations (primary and revaccinations) carried out* |
|---|---|---|---|
| 1901–02 | 90.27 | 51.90 | 352,976 |
| 1902–03 | 87.14 | 46.83 | 370,510 |
| 1903–04 | 87.20 | 54.97 | 398,634 |
| 1904–05 | 84.71 | 47.60 | 413,407 |
| 1905–06 | 90.80 | 53.25 | 489,297 |
| 1906–07 | 90.65 | 52.39 | n.a. |
| 1907–08 | 91.78 | 58.71 | n.a. |
| 1908–09 | 93.58 | 59.30 | 382,326 |
| 1909–10 | 95.27 | 61.58 | 395,444 |
| 1910–11 | 95.50 | 67.81 | 394,893 |
| 1911–12 | 96.61 | 72.77 | 507,475 |
| 1912–13 | 96.71 | 68.12 | 533,647 |
| 1913–14 | 96.59 | 65.40 | 512,801 |
| 1914–15 | 94.93 | 60.46 | 469,471 |
| 1915–16 | 97.14 | 57.18 | 459,047 |
| 1916–17 | 97.64 | 59.32 | 545,819 |
| 1917–18 | 95.88 | 49.74 | 492,008 |
| 1918–19 | 97.83 | 65.27 | 561,639 |
| 1919–20 | 97.53 | 60.58 | 839,079 |
| 1920–21 | 97.48 | 55.70 | 670,425 |
| 1921–22 | 98.07 | 58.46 | 650,140 |
| 1922–23 | 98.10 | 53.68 | 697,829 |
| 1923–24 | 98.38 | 46.76 | 752,447 |
| 1924–25 | 97.79 | 47.74 | 806,619 |
| 1925–26 | 97.81 | 42.21 | 842,729 |
| 1926–27 | 96.63 | 35.97 | 720,551 |
| 1927–28 | 92.16 | 39.88 | 870,402 |
| 1928–29 | 97.11 | 36.22 | 939,278 |
| 1929–30 | 96.75 | 34.55 | 982,645 |
| 1930–31[49] | 96.81 | 29.70 | 826,801 |

*Source*: Administration and vaccination reports for the years listed.

[49] From 1930–31, the Federated Shan States were excluded from general vaccination figures for the province.

India as the Nijland cycle or method, and sometimes as the "Java" method. The Nijland cycle involved passing the vaccine through a rabbit, then a buffalo, and finally a cow calf. The King Institute in Guindy led the way in introducing modified versions of this cycle to British India. It first replaced the buffalo with a donkey (1927), but this failed because donkeys were found to be less susceptible to the vaccine virus than buffaloes or cows. From 1930, a fourth animal was added, making the cycle a cow calf, rabbit, buffalo calf and cow calf one, which boosted both yield and potency. In 1934 and 1935, it further modified the Nijland cycle by replacing rabbits with humans. By 1929, modified versions of Nijland's method were followed all over British India, generally to maintain vaccine seed lymph potency. Meiktila's version of the Nijland cycle, which involved passing the lymph through four animals (rabbits twice, to produce a rabbit-cow calf-buffalo calf-rabbit cycle), was maintained from 1929 to the end of the 1930s.[50]

One feature that separated Meiktila from other vaccine institutes in British India and those in European colonies in Southeast Asia, especially the Dutch East Indies, was its reluctance to use dried lymph in the pre-war period. Desiccated lymph had been shown in 1902 to remain effective for five months when stored at room temperature. The two main methods of doing so for much of what remained of the colonial period were developed shortly after. In 1906, A. Carini developed a method of grinding up lymph, drying it in a vacuum, and reconstituting it in glycerine-water to destroy bacteria. Three years later, P. Achalme and Marie Phisalix dried the lymph in pieces in a vacuum, rather than grind it. In this case, the dried lymph remained effective even at a temperature of 37 degrees Celsius, offering a way of delivering it over great distances, and to hot climates. Though trials in South America and

[50] *NSVB for 1929–30*, 910; *RPHC for 1927*, 139; *RPHC for 1929*, 162, 165; *RPHC for 1930*, 242; *RPHC for 1931*, 226; *RPHC for 1932*, 194; *RPHC for 1933*, 169; *RPHC for 1934*, 170; *RPHC for 1935*, 115; *RPHC for 1936*, 181; Peter Boomgaard, "Smallpox Control in Indonesia during the Second Quarter of the Century", Paper prepared for the workshop "Local Transmutations of Global Phenomena: An Historical Reassessment of Smallpox Prevention, Vaccination and the State", The Wellcome Trust Centre for the History of Medicine at UCL, London, 30 June–1 July 2006, 6. The author would like to thank Peter Boomgaard for his generosity in sharing the paper.

Africa sometimes showed contrary results, these methods were effective enough to be adopted by France and Germany for transporting lymph to their colonies before World War I. Research in the immediate post-war years mainly demonstrated the importance of cooling before or during the drying process, and even while using dried lymph in the field. R. Wurtz and L. Camus, for example, cautioned that dried lymph had to be kept cool all the time, while it was prepared, transported, and reconstituted. They also recommended that vaccinations with it be conducted in the shade.[51]

In 1930, Meiktila conducted its own experiments with dried lymph. The dried lymph was not intended to replace most of the lymph produced at the depot, only that meant for distant and less accessible areas. Ultimately, 1,700 doses were produced and sent to stations in Mawlaik, Falam, Loimwe, Hlegu, and even the Andamans. However, its performance was poor. One reason for this was that the drying process seemed to have destroyed a significant quantity of the virus, making the dried lymph less potent than the usual preserved lymph. Another important factor was that vaccinators in Burma mixed the dried lymph with glycerine, which, it was observed, exposed it to contamination. The result was that Meiktila abandoned experiments with dried lymph, and until the depot's demise in 1942, colonial Burma made no significant use of it. Meanwhile, dried lymph made significant headway elsewhere in colonial South and Southeast Asia, producing lymph that, in one case, proved effective when tested in 1950 after being in storage for 13 years.[52]

After 1930, the momentum for research in Meiktila appears to have been spent. What had driven research was the coupling of two main factors. The first was, of course, the necessity to find the most effective lymph and to produce it at the cheapest cost. The second was the belief, held by civil surgeons throughout British India, that local conditions in their provinces, whether related to the climate, or social and cultural factors, required local solutions. Meiktila's steady improvement in lymph output had fully met the needs of the province of Burma. By 1905, after the Meiktila vaccine

[51] Collier, "The Preservation of Vaccinia Virus", 76–78.

[52] *NSVB for 1930–31*, 9; *TRVB for 1929–30 to 1931–32*, 13; *RPHC for 1934*, 170; Collier, "The Preservation of Vaccinia Virus", 78–79.

depot came into operation, Burma no longer had to depend on vaccine lymph from India or Europe. It produced enough lymph to supply all those stations not served by the Rangoon depot. In its second decade, Meiktila produced so much lymph that the Vaccination Department found that only 65 per cent of the lymph it issued in Burma was actually used. Meiktila's director was compelled to complain in 1917 about the wastage of vaccine lymph in several stations; the Mandalay municipality and Thaton district were reported to have wasted more than half the doses they were supplied. By 1932, shortly after abandoning dried lymph, Meiktila manufactured four kilograms of lymph each month, which exceeded by four times the demand in the entire province during smallpox-free years. The depot thus more than fulfilled its mandate of cultivating enough lymph that was effective for the province, reducing the need for research into new methods of ensuring its efficiency. During the 1930s, Meiktila's main energies were devoted to making lymph production more cost effective. This resulted, in the mid-1930s, in the only major change of methodology in Meiktila during the pre-war period, which was the adoption of the Malayan method of lymph production. This method required fewer cattle, thus lowering costs.[53]

The production of vaccine lymph in colonial Burma came to an end with the outbreak of World War II in the Pacific. At that time, the cultivation of lymph for the entire province was concentrated in the Meiktila vaccine depot, consisting of 14 buildings and a large staff, which had the track record of conducting some of the most innovative research in British India over three and a half decades. Meiktila had increased the annual output of vaccine lymph from 5,376 grammes or 529,189 doses in 1908–09 to 21,726 grammes or 2,105,456 doses in 1939 (the last year for reliable figures).[54] Unfortunately, the vaccine depot was destroyed in the war and never rebuilt. The brief return of the British rule after the war saw no significant efforts being made to re-establish the facility. Even after independence in 1948, rebuilding the depot for

[53] *NSVB for 1905–06*, 3; *NSVB for 1915–16*, 4; *TRVB for 1914–15 to 1916–17*, 8; *TRVB for 1917–18 to 1919–20*, 4; *RAB for 1932–33*, 96; *RAB for 1933–34*, 117; *Report on the State of Public Health in Burma during 1938*, 64.

[54] *Report on the Public Health Administration of Burma for the Year 1939*, 60; *NSVB for 1908–09*, 3.

cultivating lymph was nowhere on the agenda, and Burma once again became dependent on external sources, primarily India, for vaccine lymph.

## *Conclusion*

Overcoming the problem of ineffective vaccine lymph in a place where the hot climate, an underdeveloped intra-provincial transport system, indifferent animal health, and careless medical assistants seemed to be conspiring against it was a formidable challenge. But most of these problems were resolved with the establishment of the Meiktila vaccine depot, though not easily. Despite poor funding, problems in equipment delivery, and a range of other obstacles, repeated experiments and technical innovations led to the development of effective ways to cultivate and preserve lymph, and technologies suited to the tropical environment. As with the cultivation of animal lymph, British medical officers in Burma's vaccine depots participated in an information network that transcended colonial boundaries, and the metropole-colony divide. Often they found themselves more dependent on obtaining information about new techniques (regarding, for example, lymph rejuvenation) developed in other vaccine institutions and depots, such as in Madras or Java, than on laboratories in Europe.

One reason for this local orientation was that colonial medical officers had learnt, after years of lymph failure, that preservation techniques that worked in Europe could not simply be transplanted to the tropics. Nor was there a common answer for tropical Asia. As colonial medical officers discovered, the temperature, humidity, the availability of animals, and a range of other important conditions varied substantially within a region and even within particular provinces. Added to this were the problems of local culture and religion. All these concerns meant that medical officers had to look broadly at vaccine research activities across the region for a combination of methodologies and technologies best suited to wherever they were stationed. In the process, they became contributors to the discourse on tropical epidemiology. What the case of Burma shows is that colonial medicine can never be reduced to a simple transplanting of Western medicine. Rather, as we have seen in the case of approaches to vaccine lymph in Burma, colonial medicine represents another category of knowledge. It is informed by Western science, but the science is modified and re-exported, sometimes even rejected, on the basis of data collection, observation, experience, and local experimentation which have yielded a colonial form of "local knowledge". Although colonial medical officers might be seen to have been in the vanguard of imperial science, in actuality, many, as in the case of King and other local researchers, found themselves in opposition to the medical dogma on lymph preservation techniques, and opinions emanating from the metropole. This opposition contributed to the emergence of tropical medicine, which represented the recognition that the development of medicine had to take place in communication with local conditions.[55]

Among the many medical officers who served in the Meiktila vaccine depot, Entrican was perhaps the most important as a result of his numerous experiments to find better methods of preserving and storing the locally cultivated lymph. However, aside from the work of Entrican and other colonial medical officers, there was almost no indigenous involvement in the colonial, scientific pursuit of better lymph. Local conditions, climatic and agricultural, were all taken into consideration, but the possibility of indigenous collaboration was overlooked. Nevertheless, with the advances made in preserving lymph, the Vaccination Department finally acquired a reliable tool with which to demonstrate the efficacy and safety of vaccination. The success of the Meiktila vaccine depot and the experiments in lymph preservation raised, at least indirectly, questions about the general population's willingness to undergo vaccination. In other words, now that it was clear there was nothing wrong with the ways in which lymph was cultivated and distributed, the slow pace at which the vaccination programme was moving began to attract more attention.

55 "Local knowledge", as viewed here, differs from the practical know-how discussed by Scott in his study of the impact of authoritarian scientific modernist schemes and its displacement of indigenous local knowledge, or metis. The present study locates the main conflict not between Western and indigenous knowledge, but between metropolitan science and local experimentation and experience. For Scott's discussion see James C. Scott, *Seeing Like A State: How Certain Schemes to Improve the Human Condition Have Failed* (New Haven and London: Yale University Press, 1998), 309–41.

# 4

# *Vaccination Propaganda*

By the beginning of the twentieth century, the Vaccination Department in Burma had overcome the problem of ineffective lymph with the establishment of the Meiktila vaccine depot. While solving the lymph problem, the colonial administration also had to find ways to convince the indigenous population to accept vaccination. Vaccination propaganda developed to achieve this goal. But there was no consensus among colonial medical authorities and civil officers about how to use propaganda to promote vaccination, and their efforts often failed because of competition, contravening orders, and the confusion surrounding numerous independent efforts.

Initially, the colonial administration in British India underestimated the necessity of cultivating indigenous agency in its fight against smallpox. According to Arnold, it optimistically expected that the Indians would undertake vaccination operations on their own and that the government would then be able to take credit for introducing the procedure at little expense. When it realised the huge obstacles in the way of popular acceptance of vaccination, the medical authorities appealed to "natives of rank", such as Brahmins, urban and rural elites, and community leaders, for their support to promote vaccination. They had limited success in cities and towns such as Varanasi where Indian intellectuals, government servants, and the media backed vaccination. However, when this "top-down" strategy proved inadequate to rapidly extending vaccination, the colonial administration turned to legislation.

Bhattacharya, Harrison, and Worboys draw attention to how the issue of means of delivery divided opinion within the

An earlier version of this chapter was published in the *SOAS Bulletin of Burma Research* 4, no.1 (2006). A revised version is reproduced here with the permission of that journal.

administration. One division was between those who argued Indian volunteers who could carry out vaccination be encouraged and those who preferred more aggressive methods. The latter group was divided between those who sought laws to force Indians to accept vaccination and those who preferred "gentle and patient persuasion". This diversity of opinion on how to tackle the problem of indigenous reluctance led to the emergence of "multiple vaccinating systems" in each of the Indian presidencies.[1]

The necessity for persuasion is implied in Andrew Cunningham and Bridie Andrews's definition of "scientific medicine".

> To operate properly, scientific medicine has to take with it, or replicate abroad, its instruments and its institutions, together with its inner social hierarchies of expertise. Scientific medicine can be practised only by true believers, since it is necessary to take its thought world with one.[2]

The preventive medicine of vaccination, which many colonial medical officers believed to be "scientific medicine", thus had to be well understood, believed, and carried out. The question of how British medical authorities in Burma (and elsewhere in British India) convinced the indigenous population of the supreme efficacy of vaccination, and induced them to undergo it, is thus of critical importance to understanding the successes and failures of the colonial vaccination effort. In this effort, British civil surgeons serving in Burma frequently faced multiple predicaments, all of which were rooted in local conditions. The caste system, which was viewed as the main obstacle to vaccination in India, was absent in Burma.[3] Instead, numerous government reports allege the superstitious tendencies of a "backward" Burmese society were mainly responsible for the rejection of "modern" science. However, other reports suggest that no single factor was responsible for indigenous reluctance, and that even some of the British medical

1 Arnold, *Colonizing the Body*, 144–50. Another scholar states that the native inoculators and Brahmins were recruited to exercise their influence to gain popular support for vaccination. Deepak Kumar, "Unequal Contenders, Uneven Ground: Medical Encounters in British India, 1820–1920" in *Western Medicine as Contested Knowledge*, ed. Andrew Cunningham and Bridie Andrews, 176 (Manchester and New York: Manchester University Press, 1997); Bhattacharya, Harrison, and Worboys, *Fractured States*, 26–27.

2 Cunningham and Andrews, eds., *Western Medicine as Contested Knowledge*, 11.

3 Arnold, *Colonizing the Body*, 141–42.

authorities were non-believers in the efficacy of the operation. Scientific medicine, such as vaccination, did not speak directly to the indigenous population. The civil surgeons saw local Burmese officials, community elders, and Christian missionaries as potential agents who could play a critical role in communicating the Western knowledge about vaccination. We examine how these civil surgeons attempted to mobilise these intermediaries and the reasons they were not very successful.

In addition to the many difficulties in conveying the importance of vaccination to the indigenous population, there was disagreement between the civil surgeons in the field and the general Indian medical administration. Many civil surgeons in Burma considered publishing treatises on vaccination in the vernacular necessary. They felt so because of local experience—the Burmese in their stations did not have a clear understanding of vaccination, especially of the differences between it and variolation. Print propaganda could potentially have been the best means of spreading the message of vaccination as it was commonly held that the Burmese were the most literate of the peoples in British India because they had had the benefit of Buddhist monastic education. Nevertheless, this idea, proposed by some civil surgeons, was callously dismissed by their superiors in the colonial medical establishment. The failure to develop a consensus within the medical establishment on the advantages of print propaganda was one of the major obstacles to the spread of vaccination in the province of Burma.

## *Hearts and Minds*

Colonial vaccination reports frequently describe the Burmese as unwilling subjects. They include many stories of the failed attempts made by beleaguered medical officers to persuade the Burmese to undergo vaccination. On such officer was Wells, an assistant apothecary and Superintendent of Vaccination in Maulmain. After having spent many hours explaining the benefits of vaccination and its desirability to a group of parents, Wells found that his effort had been in vain.

> I have been fairly disgusted on being told to "come another time, as the child's or children's father is away in the jungles," or the "mother is unwell," or the "grandfather objects." . . . Others again must have the

> consent of the headman or Kyedangyee, who is either away or will not "advise." Those who ask us to "call again" contrive somehow to keep out of the way on our second visit, or the children are sent away to some relative in another street or quarter of the town.[4]

One explanation preferred by a colonial medical officer was that the Burmese were somehow resistant to change and innovation. According to Albert Fytche, the Chief Commissioner of British Burma, who wrote a general report, based on the experiences of numerous local medical officers in the 1860s, the Burmese "have little or no faith in vaccination and a certain amount of dislike to it as a dangerous innovation".[5] MacDonald, the civil surgeon in Prome, was pessimistic about winning the Burmese over to vaccination. He confided in his report to the chief commissioner, "I fear it will take many years to impress the importance of vaccination upon the Burmese, because they are so much biased against all foreign innovations."[6] The situation was the same in Upper Burma. The Burmese were accustomed to their variolation, or inoculation, using matter from human smallpox pustules, and "the Burman is very conservative in his ways and prefers his own old, though mischievous, usage to what he regards as foreign inventions".[7] In contrast, those Burmese who received an English education were believed to be more open to the practice of vaccination. It was hoped vaccination would follow English education in its spread among the Burmese.

> It is hoped that, with the spread of education, the masses of the population will be better able to appreciate the advantages of vaccination and the work of the vaccinator, which is extremely difficult in the present state of things, will be easier and less irksome.[8]

Such a process would have yielded results only in the long term and done little to prevent smallpox in the short term. So colonial medical officers had to seek other means to convince the Burmese to accept vaccination in the short term.

The limited success of early experiences, such as the Anderson experiment in Mergui in 1837, which resulted in some deaths, may

[4] *Report on Vaccination for 1868*, appendix, xxix.
[5] *RABB during 1867–68*, 167.
[6] *RVB for 1867–68*, 36–37.
[7] *NSVB for 1899–1900*, 13.
[8] *TRVB for 1896–97–1898–99*, 18.

have discouraged the Burmese from vaccinating their children. The high rate of failure because of ineffective lymph also did not serve to convince the Burmese of the procedure's efficacy. Every time a doubt arose about the safety of vaccination, it contributed to a further delay in popular acceptance of the practice. As Commissioner of Pegu R. D. Ardagh noted in 1868, it was the "want of confidence both in the system and also in the operations" that lost popular trust.[9] Even as lymph became more effective, any evidence of failure, whether real or imagined, had a significant negative effect on the progress of vaccination in the minds of the Burmese.

British medical authorities frequently pointed out indigenous officials were to be blamed for the failure of vaccination operations. Burmese officials and the local British administrative authorities were expected to support medical officers in promoting vaccination because of its inherent worth. British medical men were extremely confident about the "goodness" that vaccination would bring to the Burmese population and believed that its undeniable good conferred the moral right, and the moral obligation, on them to extend it to the Burmese. In their minds, vaccination conferred "almost perfect security against death from small-pox", and was undoubtedly "the greatest practical good" which medical science could offer.[10] To achieve this goal, they expected authorities at all levels of the colonial administration to work actively to promote the cause of vaccination.

> Government officers of all grades are expected to use their influence with the people in promoting vaccination . . . The personal influence of district officials can do a great deal to assist the department in diffusing

[9] *Report on Vaccination for 1868*, appendix, xii.

[10] *NSVB for 1899–1900*, 13. Doss, at the time serving as the civil surgeon in Akyab, also wrote, "In vain did I point out to them the advantages of successful vaccination as a prophilactic against the contagion of small-pox, and how Edward Jenner, by his patience and extraordinary genius as a Philosopher, brought into notice a prominent fact, which has driven off one of the most desolating, disfiguring, and disgusting plagues of mankind, and saved the lives of millions, and thereby multiplied the manhood of nations. Most frivolous and foolish objections were raised against the practice of vaccination at a time, when the success of the operation was almost sure, and consequently the danger of small-pox in destroying life and causing deformity may be said to be very little". *Report on Vaccination for 1868*, appendix, v.

> a knowledge of the benefits of vaccination, and in this matter the judicious use of official pressure is, it is submitted, not only legitimate, but imperative.[11]

The cooperation of local officials was considered essential for vaccination efforts because they were the ones who could bridge the gap between the medical officers and the indigenous population, using their moral influence to encourage the people to accept the practice. This was especially so in districts where variolation was more popular than vaccination. "Any determined effort" made by the officials in such places to promote vaccination was expected to have a significant effect on the success of spreading it.[12] The number of officials who provided significant help was probably small, given that those who did help received special mention in vaccination reports. One such person was the headman of Kama in Thayetmyo district who "helped popularise vaccination",[13] but such instances were rare. More frequently, the reports say the officials were not very enthusiastic. When the civil surgeon in Prome posted a public notice about the efficacy of vaccination, informing everybody that vaccinations were available in the local dispensary, the village headmen were reported to have shown the "greatest indifference in the matter".[14] Pyster, the civil surgeon in Sandoway, once accompanied the deputy commissioner because he expected the official had enough local influence to induce more Burmese children to submit to vaccination. However, an appalled Pyster noted that the official accomplished nothing. Local officials were not only indifferent to vaccination efforts, but also reportedly did more harm than good. The civil surgeon in Meiktila, for example, complained of serious irregularities on the part of some Burmese officials. He said he had found a major paradox governed the acceptance of vaccination. Burmese *myo-ouks* (town heads) were invariably two-faced, he alleged. To the medical staff, the *myo-ouk* offered his aid in promoting vaccination, but, indirectly, he was also responsible for sabotaging it and the villagers under his influence would be very much against the procedure. On the other hand, in outlying villages not under Burmese headmen,

11 *NSVB for 1899–1900*, 13.
12 *NSVB for 1911–12*, 2.
13 *TRVB for 1896–97–1898–99*, 18.
14 *RVB for 1867–68*, 36.

the civil surgeon and his vaccinators found themselves welcome, and the vaccination proceeded smoothly.[15] In Pakokku, it was reported that "the obstructive attitude of the *myo-ouk* of Myaing to an Indian Vaccinator" resulted in a decrease in the number of people who were vaccinated. This happened as long as an Indian held the post.[16] Further, British medical authorities also claimed that it was the local officials who put obstacles in the way of the vaccination effort who were the loudest in demanding it—"clamour[ing] for a vaccinator"—when smallpox actually broke out in their districts.[17]

The contradiction between colonial pride in providing free vaccinations and its unappreciated reality frustrated many civil surgeons, and led them to look down on the indigenous population. An 1868 report remarked, "To what can be attributed this neglect, but to their sheer ignorance, prejudice, and utter carelessness".[18] These feelings were strong among enthusiastic civil surgeons, such as MacDonald, who put up a large number of notices announcing vaccination schedules without much success in bringing the Burmese to the dispensaries.[19]

## *Missionaries, Languages, and Minorities*

Frustrated with the non-cooperative Burmese authorities, the government relied on another group who could exercise some influence on the indigenous population, especially in the more remote districts. Christian missionaries had established themselves as teachers and had formed bonds with the indigenous population in some, particularly minority, areas. Although British rule over parts of Burma began after the First Anglo-Burmese War (1824–26), it was only after the second war (1852) that the Western overlords began organised medical work among the indigenous population. So, for several decades, Western medicine came to Burma through medical missionaries such as Felix Carey, Adoniram Judson and his wife Anna, Jonathan Price, J. Dawson, Francis Mason, and others.

15 *Report on Vaccination for 1868*, appendix, ix; *NSVB for 1899–1900*, 13.
16 *NSVB for 1897–98*, 1.
17 *NSVB for 1899–1900*, 13.
18 *Report on Vaccination for 1868*, appendix, v.
19 Ibid., xxi.

The strategy of using the medical missionary to gain popularity among the indigenous population, and to encourage them to change their faith, did not take root until the mid-nineteenth century in British India. When medical missionary activities gradually expanded over the next half-century, they took advantage of the improvements that had come about in modern medicine. However, in Burma, Christian missionaries had begun medical activities even before the Missionary Convention of 1853 approved the use of medical work as a means of evangelisation. A pioneer was Carey, who introduced vaccination to Burma in 1811. He arrived in Rangoon at the end of 1807 after staying in Bengal and translating the New Testament into Sanskrit, Oriya, Hindi, Marathi, and Punjabi. Surprisingly, the introduction of vaccination was reported to have been a success. Carey's subjects for vaccination were the European residents in Rangoon, but it did not take long for the indigenous population to begin showing an interest in this new medical practice. One Burmese *myo-wun* (governor), after witnessing the successful vaccination of another person's child, asked that his own children be vaccinated. He also requested Carey to provide him with more information on cowpox and vaccination. When he was satisfied with the explanation, he had the nine main members of his household vaccinated despite the opposition of his wife. They included men, women, and children, and the wife was reportedly later satisfied with the result.[20] News about the new preventive measure circulated among the Burmese elite and Carey soon attracted the court's attention. He was summoned to treat a sick prince, but the would-be patient died before Carey left Rangoon for the capital, Ava, and the trip was cancelled.

The Burmese court maintained an interest in Western medical practices. In 1813, King Bodawhpaya (ruled 1782–1819) again summoned Carey to vaccinate his grandson, the crown prince and

[20] Rosemary Fitzgerald, "'Clinical Christianity': The Emergence of Medical Work as a Missionary Strategy in Colonial India, 1800–1914", Biswamoy Pati and Mark Harrison, eds., *Health, Medicine, and Empire: Perspectives on Colonial India* (New Delhi: Orient Longman, 2001), 97–102; Maung Shwe Wa, Genevieve and Erville Sowards, *Burma Baptist Chronicle* (Rangoon: University Press, 1963), 145; B. R. Pearn, "Felix Carey and the English Baptist Mission to Burma", *Journal of Burma Research Society* 28 (1938), 12–13,16.

future king Ba-gyì-daw (1819–37). Though Carey did not at the time possess vaccine, the Burmese court paid him great respect, bringing him "in a 'golden boat' in the character of 'Rajah Sippey' or Royal Doctor, and offering him 'a gold medal and a title' and 'Burmese dress'". To maintain his amicable relationship with the court, Carey obtained vaccine from Calcutta in 1814. However, his diary is silent about whether it was used on the crown prince. The Indian medical board paid special attention to Carey's success in introducing vaccination to Burma and the royal court. Russell, the Superintendent General of Vaccination in the Bengal Presidency, noted,

> He [has] carried with him [to the Burmese court] supplies of Virus in all forms, and I hope soon to be able to submit to the Board the successful result of his . . . exertions, to give éclat to the practice in a Country where the Influence of Rank and Station . . . be so great.[21]

Besides Carey, there were other Western missionaries whose medical skills were availed of by the court in Ava.[22]

Despite the Indian government's excitement over the successful introduction of vaccination, the Burmese court was never fully converted to it. A Burmese chronicle refers to three princesses who were inoculated in the court in 1883 after smallpox had already become a threat.

> Among the four royal princesses, three of them except for the second royal princess were inoculated. They developed smallpox and did not recover well from the attack. The royal physician and the Italian doctor summoned the distinguished *Beindaw hsaya* and *Dats hsaya* from the inner and outer quarters of the golden royal capital to the royal audience hall, and they discussed their remedies and gave treatment.[23]

[21] IOR/F/4/11883, Report of the Superintendent General of Vaccination for the Year 1813, "The exertions of Mr Carey, a missionary and others favourably noticed", Extract from the Public Letter from Bengal, Calcutta, 27 July 1814, OIOC.

[22] For example, one missionary called Ignatius performed medical duties in Ava for the court. "Extracts of Letters from Rev A Judson to Rev G. H. Hough Now at Serampore. January 22, 1821", *American Baptist Missionary Magazine* 3, no. 7 (1822), 256.

[23] U Tin (Mandalay), comp., *Kon-baung-zet-maha-ya-zawin-daw-gyi* (Rangoon: Leidi Mangain, 1967), 3: 634. The translation is the author's.

Before the 1850s, Western missionaries were able to introduce vaccination for brief periods in Burma, often in isolated localities. However, they did not have the resources to persevere with the practice for a length of time, or cover broad sweeps of territory. This was especially true of Upper Burma, where the missionaries did not generally have the support of the royal court or its permission to reach out to the Buddhist population. There is also no evidence that the Burmese court tried to use its authority to support vaccination efforts by missionaries among the general population.

The introduction of vaccination to the population at large, and on a more permanent basis, depended on vaccination becoming a concern of the state, which happened in Burma only in areas under British rule. With government support came government supplies of lymph for missionary vaccinators, who had a stronger presence in the hill areas among Christianised minorities than the small colonial administration. This aid was forthcoming also because the colonial government realised that it needed the assistance of missionaries for its vaccination efforts. The realisation was based on the observation of many civil surgeons that the spread of smallpox depended on the movement of people, and this meant fighting the disease throughout the province, not just in areas under their immediate supervision.

When government vaccinators attempted to extend vaccination to areas populated by minority groups, they found missionary aid critical. In the initial years, vaccinators accompanied missionaries to Karen villages in the hope, apparently realised, that the evangelists would use their influence to convince the population to accept vaccination. For example, in 1868, the Reverend Justis Brainard Vinton agreed to take a vaccinator with him to the Karen and Shan districts where many villagers had become Christians. It was reported that 3,575 people were successfully vaccinated on this tour despite the opposition of "certain petty Government Burmese Officials".[24] As the author of the "Report on the Practice of Vaccination in the Town and Suburbs of Rangoon for the Year 1867–68", commented, "Had it not been for the Christian religion, which prevails in these Districts, the result would have been far otherwise".[25] In this particular case, Vinton planned to visit

[24] *RVB for 1867–68*, 14.
[25] Ibid., 16.

Pegu, taking two vaccinators with him to continue operations. However, illness prevented this. On learning of Vinton's poor health, Sub-assistant Surgeon N. M. Bhuttacherjee in Rangoon lamented, "We thereby lost the opportunity of extending Vaccination to the District of Pegu. There, perhaps, this operation was never introduced except through missionary labour".[26] This was probably an exaggeration. Nevertheless, Vinton's reputation did have a huge influence in persuading the indigenous population to undergo vaccination. In 1868, the vaccination report for Rangoon recorded that a majority of the 5,672 people vaccinated were Shans and Karens. They reportedly accepted vaccination because "one of the vaccinators . . . accompanied [the] American Missionary, the Reverend Mr Vinton, on a journey to the Eastern frontier".[27]

Despite the great popularity of Christian missionaries among a few, though substantial, minority groups such as the Shans and Karens, the missionaries themselves acknowledged that they had yet to extend their influence among the Burman majority. It was reported that Christianity would enlighten the "ignorant" Burmans, helping them to benefit from the benevolence of the West, and adopt the preventive measure of vaccination. Mason attempted to carry out this task through a project to publish his medical text in the Burmese language.

## *Mason and his Medical Book*

Mason (1799–1874) was the first missionary to attempt publishing a description of vaccination in Burmese. In doing so, he contributed to a slow stream of early efforts to bring Western medical knowledge, including the "gift" of vaccination, to the Burmese. He was preceded in this by Henry Burney and an unnamed Burmese Catholic priest in the 1830s. Mason had been appointed by the Baptist Missionary Board to join fellow missionary George Dana Boardman in Tavoy in January 1831, shortly before the latter's death. He continued to work there until 1852, when he was assigned to the Toungoo and Karen hill areas, "newly opened" during the Second Anglo-Burmese War. There he put himself to work translating and publishing Western medical works in Sgau

[67] Ibid., 14.

[27] *Report on Vaccination for 1868*, 15.

and Bghai Karen, and also became known as a very strong advocate of providing education in vernacular languages. He initially produced Sgau and Bghai Karen editions of his *Materia Medica*, following them up with another *Materia Medica* in Burmese, which was three times the size of the earlier works.[28]

Mason and the colonial government found it useful to cooperate in this project, and, in December 1866, he requested that the government pay 1,000 rupees to subsidise publishing 2,000 copies of the Burmese text, which had been finished under the title of *Hseì-hnín-a-gyaùng-sa*. The aim was to sell the book at an affordable eight annas per copy,[29] and the British government agreed to provide the funds on the recommendation of Horace Spearman, the officiating secretary to Captain D. Hildebrand, the officiating secretary to the chief commissioner of British Burma. Spearman argued, "The work is likely to be of great value to the Burmese people, with whom, medicine, as an art is mixed up with astrology and the practice of charms".[30] In exchange for funding, the government required Mason to allow it to buy 1,000 copies of the book for it to distribute.[31] The government side of this project was never taken up. The Education Department did purchase 500 copies of Mason's

28 Shwe Wa, *Burma Baptist Chronicle*, 87, 115–16; 1/1 (A) Accession 1374, 1867–68, File no. 442 "Mason's Materia Medica", Box 1868 (19), Letter from Horace Spearman, Officiating Secretary, to Captain C. D. Hildebrand, Officiating Secretary to the Chief Commissioner, British Burma, to the Secretary to the Government of India, Home Department, dated Rangoon, 20 February 1867, NAUM, 4.

29 1/1 (A) Accession 1374, 1867–68, File no. 442 "Mason's Materia Medica", Box 1868 (19), Letter from Horace Spearman, Officiating Secretary, to Captain C. D. Hildebrand, Officiating Secretary to the Chief Commissioner, British Burma, to the Secretary to the Government of India, Home Department, dated Rangoon, 20 February 1867, NAUM; Sò-myín-hnín and Twet-aung, *Amyò-tha-yè-hnín-Myanmá-hsèi-binya-shin-myà* (Rangoon: Sapeibiman, 1998), 217. Also, there seems to have been a different version of this text—Rev Mason, *A Burmese Hand-book of Medicine* (Toungoo: Karen Institute Press, 1866).

30 Ibid.

31 1/1 (A) Accession 1374, 1867–68, File no. 442 "Mason's Materia Medica", Box 1868 (19), Letter from Horace Spearman, Officiating Secretary, to Captain C. D. Hildebrand, Officiating Secretary to the Chief Commissioner, British Burma, to the Secretary to the Government of India, Home Department, dated Rangoon, 20 February 1867, f. 4.

medical text, but they were not put to good use—"These books are now lying idle in the Director's Office, a circumstance which, considering the usefulness of the books, is much regretted".[32]

Disappointed at the lack of government enthusiasm, Mason distributed some copies to Buddhist monks, who, he assumed, presumably because of his own intimate knowledge of the close relationship between religious men and their communities, would have the greatest influence among the general, Buddhist, population. It is not clear whether Mason's intention was to use the monks and their influence to get the population to accept Western medicine, thus opening the back door for Christian proselytisation. However, he certainly believed that it would encourage the Burmese to begin to accept changes that bettered their condition in general. He said,

> Most of the Burmese priests practice medicine to a greater or less extent; and I always find a copy of this book an acceptable present to them, and were the book distributed in the *khyoungs*, it could not but contribute materially to promote the interests of monastic education, which the Government is now endeavouring to improve in accordance with the plans of the late Chief Commissioner. It replaces astrology and charms with tried remedies and scientific antidotes.[33]

Mason did gain support from some monks, and, after a while, some of them began to come to him for medicines they had read about in his medical book.[34]

The most important aspect of Mason's *Materia Medica*, however, is that it provides one of the first descriptions of Western vaccination in Burmese. Translated into English, the Burmese text of the entry on vaccination in the 1868 edition reads,

> Vaccination. To inject cowpox. In English, it is called vaccination. The person who receives an injection of cowpox develops only minor fever. Pain also [lasts] 10 days. Within 12 days, [the pain] vanishes. The body does not ache either. There will be no [development of] pox matter also. People who receive a definite injection with pus and develop fever later do not develop pox or pain. [They are] freed [from smallpox]. Some people receive an [incomplete] insertion of cowpox pus, and after that, while thinking that they have immunity, they develop smallpox again. Although there were some who developed [smallpox] again, they

32 *Report on Public Instruction in British Burma for the Year 1872–73* (Rangoon: Government Press), 70.

33 Ibid.

34 Ibid.

> amounted to very few [cases] among many people. Those who catch smallpox naturally and those who receive pox [types] from other people might develop smallpox again. Although one develops smallpox again after completing [an injection] of cowpox matter, the pain is mild. The fever is also minimal. There are not so many pocks. It is also not so bad. It will also not be long. No one will die. According to the English medical doctors' observations, out of six people who catch smallpox naturally, one will likely die [a one in six mortality rate]. As for those who get an injection of smallpox matter taken from another person, one in 200 will likely die. As for those who get an injection of cowpox matter, only one in 100,000 will likely die. Before the injection of cowpox matter from the cow was found, in Western countries, among all adults and children who [were] treated, one out of 10 died of smallpox. Now, there were fewer people who die from smallpox. Thinking about [one] place, in Toungoo town where a small number of people live, smallpox visited them every year. However, for 10 years, in Hastwe, a Kayin village near Toungoo, no case of smallpox has occurred. If someone asks why, it is because many of the villagers have already had vaccination. Thus, they are free from natural smallpox. When doctors conduct vaccination operations, whenever there are small children who have not had smallpox, let them be vaccinated.[35]

Mason's description was incorporated and expanded in a later work by a Burmese author, *hsaya* Tout. This 1881 work, *Ingalei-hseì-kyan* ("The Handbook of English Medicine"), was perhaps the most important secular work on Western medicine for the Burmese in the late nineteenth century.[37] Although some sentences were modified, in some cases to correct Mason's grammar (in some instances, subject and object markers are reversed with the subject and object respectively), and some new sentences added, the impact of his contribution could be seen in the numerous sentences drawn verbatim, or nearly so, from his text. And the overall structure of the description remained the same. Rendered into English, *hsaya* Tout's Burmese entry reads,

> The method of injecting cowpox, vaccination, [is conducted] in order to save many people from the very scary smallpox. The people of

35 Mason, *A Burmese Hand-book of Medicine,* 59–60. The translation is the author's.

36 *Hsaya* Tout, *Ingalei-hseì-kyan* (Rangoon: Bengalee Job Printing Press, 1881). This work is also included in the list of important early Burmese works on Western medicine by So Myint and Tout Aung in *Amyò-tha-yè-hnín-Myanmá-hsèi-binya-shin-myà*, 217.

> Myanmar [Burma] knew a little about the method of the doctors of Western medicine for more than 50 years. This method is to take pus matter from a cow's wound first, and then cut the person's skin with a small knife and insert (pus) into it. The English people call this method vaccination. This method leaves only a little scar on the arm. [The person who receives vaccination] develops only a minor fever. The wound will also vanish within 10 to 12 days. The body does not ache either. One does not have to suffer. People who receive a definite injection with pus and develop fever do not later develop pox or pain. Some people who develop symptoms received an [incomplete] insertion of cowpox pus, and after that, while thinking that they have immunity, they develop smallpox again. Although there were some who developed [smallpox] again, they amounted to very few [cases] among many people. Those who caught smallpox naturally and those who received pox [types] from other people might develop smallpox again. Although one sometimes develops smallpox again after completing [an injection] of cowpox matter, the pain is mild. The fever is also minimal. There are no pocks. According to the English medical doctors' observations, out of six people who catch smallpox naturally, one will likely die [a one in six mortality rate]. As for those who get an injection of smallpox matter taken from another person, one in two hundred will likely die. As for those who get an injection of cowpox matter, no one will die out of 100,000. Before the injection of cowpox matter from the cow was found, in Western countries, among all adults and children who [were] treated, one out of ten died of smallpox. Now, there are few people who die from smallpox. Those who have scars are also rare. Among the people in Burma, many have died from the frightening smallpox malady every year. In [our] country, three will likely die out of every five people who develop smallpox. That is the way it is. Do the same thing as the Western country. Try to use the method of vaccination.[37]

Though they had cooperated to publish Mason's work, which described vaccination in Burmese, helped each other out in obtaining good lymph, and visited villages together, the government officials and missionaries diverged in their approaches to spreading the word about vaccination by the end of 1868. While Mason's work continued to influence Burmese writers into the twentieth century, civil surgeons struggled to produce their own treatise, apparently unaware of, or unwilling to acknowledge, the American missionary's influential work.

[37] Tout, *Ingalei-hseì-kyan*, 138–39. The translation is the author's.

## Medicine, Language and Treatises

While missionaries in Burma had early success in making use of local languages and concentrated their efforts in religion (and medicine) mainly on the non-Burman minorities, their British government counterparts did the opposite. Lacking numbers, the British administration in colonial Burma concentrated its attention on the lowlands, which were dominated by the main Burman ethnic group, and learnt Burmese, the lingua franca of the region, if they learnt a local language at all.

There was a wide chasm between the Government of India's recognition that it was important for medical officials to learn the indigenous language and actually getting them to learn it. Even before the beginning of British government vaccination efforts in Burma, that is, before the government took over East India Company lands in Burma in 1858, the problem of communication between company medical authorities and the indigenous population had emerged. Language was recognised as one of the key issues affecting medical work in Burma. Naturally, this should have meant a strong effort on the part of the government to encourage its medical officers to learn Burmese. However, the East India Company left a legacy of institutional rules and practices that took time to sort out. On 18 March 1854, for example, the East India Company Governor General issued orders that medical officers should pass an examination in the colloquial language of the indigenous population to qualify to be in charge of a jail hospital (the main station for medical officers in India and Burma in the mid-nineteenth century). Otherwise, the company could terminate the medical officer's appointment.[38] However, the medical officers serving in Burma cleverly circumvented the language requirement by claiming that their ability in Hindi fulfilled the condition, since, in India, of which British Burma was now a part, Hindi was the major colloquial language. In 1858, Commissioner Phayre, who was in charge of the qualifying examination in Hindi, attempted to allay Calcutta's fears that medical officers in Burma had not observed

[38] 1/1 (A) Accession no. 399, 1858, File no. 73, "Examination of Medical Officers in Colloquial Burmese", Box 1858 (3), Letter to the Secretary to the Government of India, Foreign Department, dated Rangoon, 28 June 1858, NAUM.

the 1854 order by confirming that all the medical officers at the jail hospital in Pegu had passed the colloquial Hindustani examination. This apparent circumvention of the order drew severe criticism from British officials in India. R. B. Chapman, the officiating Under Secretary to the Government of India, complained in response to a letter from Phayre,

> It is mentioned that all the other Medical Officers in charge of jails have passed the colloquial examination in Hindustani, whereby the letter of the Hon'ble Court's orders is observed, though not the spirit, as a knowledge of Hindoostani will not enable Medical men to converse with their Burmese patients.[39]

To prevent further attempts to get around the rules, the Governor General specified that all medical officers pass a colloquial examination in Burmese to qualify for appointment in the jail hospital in Pegu.[40] Phayre's response indicates the significance accorded by early British administrators to government medical efforts in Burma was rather superficial, something that would hamper real reform in the vaccination effort until the 1880s. He complained to the Indian government,

> I have the honour to report for the information of his Honour in Council, that with the exception of the Jails at Rangoon and Bassein, all the Jails in the Province are under the charge of Medical Officers who hold these situations only temporarily, in as long as the Regiments of Establishment of Troops to which they may belong happens to be quartered at the stations, and I apprehend that some difficulty would be experienced if such officers were required to pass in Burmese.[40]

The Indian government was convinced that, nonetheless, medical officers in Burma should be able to converse in Burmese with their patients—to understand the Burmese and, perhaps more importantly, to make themselves understood to the Burmese. The

39 1/1 (A) Accession no. 399, 1858, File no. 73, "Examination of Medical Officers in Colloquial Burmese", Box 1858 (3), Letter from R. B. Chapman, Esquire, Officiating Under Secretary to the Government of India, to Major Arthur Phayre, Commisioner of Pegue, dated 6 August 1858, NAUM.

40 Ibid.

41 1/1 (A) Accession no. 399, 1858, File 73, "Examination of Medical Officers in Colloquial Burmese in Pegu", Box 1858 (3), Letter to [Cecil Beaden] the Secretary to the Government of India, Officiating in the Foreign Department, Fort William, dated Rangoon, 31 August 1858, NAUM.

government ordered Phayre, despite his reservations, to draw up rules for a colloquial Burmese examination after the latter explained that "no specific rules have ever been laid down for the examination of officers in the Burmese colloquial only."[42] Indeed, the problem of the language competence of British medical officers in Burma came to the attention of the Indian government after Phayre tried to recommend that John Davis, the medical officer in Bassein, be deemed to have passed the language examination though he had taken no exam. As proof of the doctor's competence in Burmese, he offered the testimony of the deputy commissioner in Bassein, who confirmed that Davis was both able to understand his patients and make himself understood to them in Burmese. But he had no proof of the deputy commissioner's ability in colloquial Burmese, and thus his competence to testify how good Davis was with the language.[43] Phayre's plan for the language examination was to have committees consisting of two officers who had passed the examination in Burmese. They would ask questions and translate examinees' responses, and a medical officer would aid in constructing 15 or 16 sentences which were likely to come up in conversation between a doctor and a patient. The questions would be read slowly and the examiners would make certain that successful candidates could respond with "readiness, correctness of idiom and tolerable accuracy of grammar".[44]

By the 1880s, more attempts were made in Burma to circulate correct information about vaccination among the indigenous population. This may have been influenced by a similar effort that was being made on the subcontinent by the colonial medical authorities there.[45] In Burma, civil surgeons undertook independent

42 1/1 (A) Accession no. 399, 1858, File 73, "Examination of Medical Officers in Colloquial Burmese", Box 1858 (3), Letter to the Secretary to the Government of India, Foreign Department, dated Rangoon, 28 June 1858, NAUM.

43 Ibid.

44 1/1 (A) Accession no. 399, 1858, File 73, "Examination of Medical Officers in Colloquial Burmese in Pegu", Box 1858 (3), Attachment to Phayre, Letter to Cecil Beadon, Secretaty to the Government of India, Officer to Foreign Department, Fort William, dated Rangoon, 25 August 1858, NAUM.

45 Bhattacharya, Harrison, and Worboys mention a pamphlet for "popular information" about vaccination prepared by Edmondston Charles, the Superintendent General of Vaccination, India. He included a chart

efforts to raise awareness about vaccination. A civil surgeon in Rangoon, for example, in 1864, issued invitations in public journals, in both English and Burmese, requesting everyone to come to his dispensary to be vaccinated or, rather, to "receive what the genius of Jenner provided for them". He said, "For not being vaccinated . . . at least in Rangoon, no one can have any excuse".[46] In late 1867, an advertisement for vaccination was published in both English and Burmese in the local newspaper.[47] In Prome, public notices were posted in Burmese in an effort to notify the general population of the availability of vaccination and its efficacy. However, this did not improve the vaccination rate—"Not a single case was brought nor the slightest attention paid to the notice".[48]

Simple advertisements and notices on vaccination proved to have no effect in convincing the indigenous population to accept the practice. A. Callaway Nisbet was the most vocal advocate of publishing and circulating treatises explaining vaccination in the vernacular. His suggestion was based on the years of experience he had as a civil officer in several districts in British Burma. He had officiated as the civil surgeon in Akyab, replacing then Assistant Surgeon Cowie, as well as covered for the medical leave of Sub-assistant Surgeon Kellie Coorman Huthe from December 1862 to May 1863. On 29 May 1863, he was appointed the civil surgeon in Bassein, replacing the sickly Davis who died just after he had asked for medical leave.[49] The station in Bassein involved Nisbet

comparing vaccination and inoculation, and indicating that vaccination was safer than inoculation. Bhattacharya, Harrison, and Worboys, *Fractured States*, 56–57.

46 *Report on the Health of the Indigenous Peoples of British Burma, and on the Supposed Causes of the Sparseness of the Population in that Province* (Rangoon: Rangoon Times Press, 1864), 41.

47 *RVB for 1867–68*, 15.

48 Ibid., 22.

49 1/1(A) Accession 612, 1863, 49 "Apptt. Of Asstt. Surgeon A. J. Cowie as Civil Surgeon at Rangoon in the Room of Asstt. Surgeon J. E. Dickenson resigned", Box 1863 (2), Letter from Davies, Secretary to Chief Commissioner, British Burma and Agent to Colonel Durand, dated Rangoon, 6 January 1863, NAUM, 5–6; 1/1 (A) Accession 612, 1863, 49 "Apptt. Of Asstt. Surgeon A. J. Cowie as Civil Surgeon at Rangoon in the Room of Asstt. Surgeon J. E. Dickenson resigned", Box 1863 (2), Letter from Davies, Secretary to Chief Commissioner, British Burma, to the Officiating Secretary to the

in vaccination and other health matters because he was in charge of the local dispensary as well as the town jail.

While practising vaccination in Akyab and Bassein, Nisbet faced difficulties in getting people to turn up for vaccination. In 1865, he put his mind to solving this problem and came up with the idea of writing a brief treatise on vaccination and variolation in the Burmese language for circulation among the indigenous population.[50] Though he apparently sketched out such a treatise, it was neither printed nor published, and went uncirculated among the Burmese. References to it in official reports and correspondence indicate that he either discussed his ideas with his peers and superiors, or circulated a draft of the treatise among them, or both. From 1865, Nisbet was persistent in advocating the circulation of such a treatise in Burmese. In a letter to Charles Planck, Inspector General of Prisons, he expressed his frustration, "I have repeatedly but unsuccessfully advocated the plan referred to in the remarks of the Governor General in Council to which my attention is directed".[51]

Nisbet's planck for improving the indigenous response to vaccination in Burma by circulating treatises were complicated by his rigorous approach to all aspects of the vaccination effort under his supervision. In fact, he became so persistent that he appears to have been considered a nuisance by some of his superiors. He criticised the government for not making vaccination compulsory in Burma as well as for not prosecuting inoculators who were harming the official campaign.[52] Perhaps due to Nisbet's criticism of the government, Chief Commissioner Albert Fytche seemed to have an unfavourable impression of him.

---

Government of India, dated Rangoon, 9 July 1863, NAUM, 7–9; 1/1 (A) Accession 614, 1863, File no. 4, "Grant of leave to Dr J. Davis, Surgeon of Bassein", Box 1863 (2), Letter from the Secretary to the Governor General of India to Chief Commissioner, British Burma, Simla, 26 June 1863, NAUM, 8.

50 *RVB for 1867–68*, 45.

51 1/1 (A) Accession 1083, 1867–68, 5 (2) "Treatise on Vaccination in the Vernacular", Box 1868 (1), Letter from A. C. Nisbet, Superintendent, Bassein Jail, to the Charles Planck, Inspector General of Prisons, dated Bassein, 20 December 1867, NAUM, 64.

52 *RVB for 1867–68*, 23.

> Dr Nisbet seems to have a morbid fear of incorrect returns, a fear laudable in itself, but most pernicious when carried to such an extent as seems to have been done in this case, bringing vaccination almost to a stop in one of the most important towns and districts of the province.[53]

Government annoyance with Nisbet, which is evident in this and other correspondence, may have influenced the medical authorities' response to his "treatise" plan.[54] However, among his peers, the other civil surgeons in stations in British Burma, he could count on a good deal of support. Like him, they faced seemingly insurmountable obstacles, and were probably able to understand his "crusade", even if they did not emulate him. Many medical officers, for example, began requesting that some sort of advertisement on the efficacy of vaccination be circulated in the vernacular. MacDonald, the civil surgeon in Prome, supported Nisbet's plan, "I am of opinion that circulating treatises in the vernacular would be more likely than any other to bring about so desirable a result".[55] John W. T. Whitaker, the civil surgeon in Tavoy, was more precise in his request even though the plan had not been finalised. He requested that "a few hand-sheets in Burmese" be forwarded to his station.[56] Likewise, W. Miller, the civil surgeon in Thayetmyo, requested that "one thousand copies in Burmese . . . be forwarded to [him] for distribution".[57]

53 *RABB during 1867–68*, 166–67.

54 Nisbet's outspoken "exactitude" led to problems with non-government authorities as well. He complained, for example, of the cold shoulder given him by "the editor of a local and influential medical journal". He also related that these medical authorities "completely ignored the fact in an acrimonious criticism of my vaccination report for 1866–67 and that with reference to an Epidemic constitution naturally existing and more over superintended by the most unheard of abuse of the practice of inoculation vide *Indian Medical Gazette* of the 1st August 1867, page 204 which the Editor declined to publish my reply". 1/1 (A) Accession 1083, 1867–68, 5 (2) "Treatise on Vaccination in the Vernacular", Box 1868 (1), Letter from A. C. Nisbet, Superintendent, Bassein Jail, to Charles Planck, Inspector General of Prisons, dated Bassein, 20 December 1867, NAUM, 64–65.

55 *RVB for 1867–68*, 36–37.

56 Ibid, 52.

57 1/1 (A) Accession 1083, 1867–68, 5 (2) "Treatise on Vaccination in the Vernacular" Box 1868 (1), Letter from Dr W. Miller, Civil Surgeon, Thayet-myo, to Commissioner of Pegu, dated Rangoon, 21 February 1868, NAUM, 48.

There was a growing consensus among the civil surgeons in Burma that the different points Nisbet wanted to be included in the treatise were important enough to be made. These points, in Nisbet's own words, were (1) "the peculiar advantages of vaccination according to the best medical authorities"; (2) "the precautions necessary for its complete success"; (3) "the result which had rewarded the operation wherever fairly employed"; and (4) "what might be reasonably expected of it in this country if it were allowed fair play".[58] Other civil surgeons in Burma began to contribute to the growing discourse on the "little" treatise. For example, many felt that, in addition to these points, it was necessary to inculcate the notion of "the prophylactic", or preventive medicine, among the indigenous population. This idea was generally absent in the Burmese understanding of medicine. Unless a clear, external, and imminent danger, such as the outbreak of an epidemic, began to threaten their lives, the Burmese were averse to vaccination. Charles R. G. Parker, for example, reported in 1867 that the outbreak of measles, chickenpox and minor smallpox caused a minor panic among the people in Toungoo. Waves of Burmese people rushed to get their children vaccinated. However, once the panic died down, no children were brought to the dispensaries. There was no mistaking the disinterest—even placards "put up in various parts of the Town giving the day and hour for attendance" attracted nobody now that the crisis was over. However, Parker said, "I did not think that Burmese had any special aversion to vaccination".[59] Rather, he considered them "lethargic". This feeling was shared by other civil surgeons, and they considered it essential that the indigenous population be educated about the prophylactic advantage of vaccination. Sub-Assistant Surgeon and Superintendent of Vaccination Doss advised, "Treatises on the advantages of vaccination as a prophylactic against the contagion of small pox in the vernacular should be circulated freely among all classes of people that are able to read".[60]

58 1/1(A) Accession 1083, 1867–68, 5 (2) "Treatise on Vaccination in the Vernacular", Box 1868 (1), Letter from A. C. Nisbet, Superintendent, Bassein Jail, to Charles Planck, Inspector General of Prisons, dated Bassein, 20 December 1867, NAUM, 64–65.

59 *RVB for 1867–68*, 41–42.

60 Ibid., 4.

Some civil surgeons also observed that there was the need to end the confusion between vaccination and variolation in the popular mind. They argued that colonial medical authorities had failed to satisfactorily differentiate between the two procedures. Pyster, for example, reported that the Burmese erroneously believed that vaccination and variolation were the same thing.[61] To emphasise the difference, some civil surgeons suggested that the advantages of vaccination over variolation be mentioned. P. George Paul, Superintendent of Vaccination in Myanaung, commented,

> I also think that this all-important subject should be more prominently made to engage the attention of the people by means of printed tracts (one side English and the other Burmese) containing a few particulars of advantages of Vaccination over inoculation.[62]

Nisbet urged the launch of such an advertisement campaign as soon as possible so that the Burmese would abandon their prejudice and accept vaccination before smallpox broke out again and caused many avoidable deaths.[63] While he and other civil surgeons continued to push the government to accept their plan, some of the authorities did not consider it essential. They believed that the best advertisement for vaccination was successful vaccination itself and insisted that demonstrating how effective vaccination was would be far more productive than any other form of propaganda. John McNeale Donnelly, Superintendent of Vaccination for British Burma, reacted to Paul's support for the treatise by commenting, "I should think that the wonderful success that has attended his labours must have taught the people of Myan-oung a deeper lesson than any we can hope to inculcate by means of persuasive essays".[64] Further examining the true obstacles to vaccination, Donnelly admitted that "there might be a good reason" unsuccessful vaccines were persuading some people not to undergo vaccination, but this number would remain relatively small. In truth, ineffective vaccination, he believed, would appear to nullify

[61] *Report on Vaccination for 1868*, appendix, ix.

[62] Ibid., xix.

[63] 1/1(A) Accession 1083, 1867–68, 5 (2) "Treatise on Vaccination in the Vernacular", Box 1868 (1), Letter from A. C. Nisbet, Superintendent, Bassein Jail, to Charles Planck, Inspector General of Prisons, dated Bassein, 20 December 1867, NAUM, 64–65.

[64] *Report on Vaccination for 1868*, 16.

the British promise of lifetime immunity to the scourge of smallpox, but at least 95 per cent of those in whom vaccination failed would still believe that they had gained immunity. This faith in the success of the operation, he implied, was due to the magnitude of the sacrifice made by the average Burmese for immunity "which was promised him as the reward of his moral courage in departing from the usage of his country, and setting at defiance the contingent ridicule of his friends, as well as the prompting of his own apathy".[65] Donnelly thus argued that propaganda was unnecessary, for the Burmese would remain blissfully ignorant of the faults of vaccination and most would eventually accept it if the civil surgeons were not "over anxious" to obtain immediate acceptance.[66]

Despite the government's effort to reject Nisbet's plan, Colonel D. Brown, the Commissioner of the Tenasserim division, reluctantly began to discuss sanctioning it. However, it is clear that government officials were trying to minimise the influence of the treatise. Brown wrote,

> I consider that it will not be necessary to go to the expense of printing the treatise in more languages than one, and that should be Burmese, which is more generally in use than any other language, while the advantages of vaccination are clearly stated, the danger of inoculation should be dwelt on in the treatise. The circulation of a short treatise in Burmese would I believe sate the curiosity of the people. It would draw their attention to vaccination and would probably increase the number of applicants for the operation.[67]

The government, though moving slowly and always attempting to avoid undue expense, eventually began to support the treatise plan, but with strings attached. Rather than allow civil surgeons to dictate the government's vaccination policy, the authorities attempted to keep the project small and assume control over its details. In March 1868, the deputy commissioner of Tavoy and the commissioner of Maulmain attempted to modify the content of the treatise on the point that vaccination was more advantageous than

65 Ibid., 9.

66 Ibid.

67 1/1 (A) Accession 1083, 1867–1868, File no. 5 (2) "Treatises on Vaccination in the Vernacular", Box 1868 (1), Letter from Colonel D. Brown, Commissioner of Tenasserim Division, British Burma, to Horace Spearman, Esquire, Officiating Assistant Secretary to the Chief Commissioner, dated 4 February 1868, NAUM, 7–8.

variolation. They suggested that there was no need to emphasise this, since variolation was practised only when smallpox broke out and the Burmese always feared it tended to spread smallpox.[68] Their intention seems to have been to indirectly minimise the influence of the treatise. The authorities also exerted control over the form in which the treatise would be written, translated, and published. Rather than publish Nisbet's 1865 treatise as presented, Planck, the Inspector General of Prisons, suggested in an April 1868 letter to the chief commissioner that the treatise should be concise and composed by "the best Burmese scholar in the Province". Nisbet could have some involvement, if the government thought it necessary, and provide a brief statement on the subject that could be used by the Burmese scholar for information and guidance.[69] However, Nisbet's original treatise would not be used, or perhaps even seen, and the new treatise would be written independently and published directly in Burmese, circumventing possible interference by the civil surgeons.

Nisbet—and presumably his fellow civil surgeons—remained defiant and pursued an independent plan. Less than a year after the government began to attempt to remodel his original plan, he published his own "short" treatise on vaccination, translated into vernacular Burmese and Sgau Karen, in February 1869. Since he could not depend on official support—and possibly even fearing the heavy hand of the government if he did not act quickly—Nisbet took the treatise directly to the public through the Catholic press and the newspapers. He received plenty of help from an old friend, Father S. DeCruz of the Roman Catholic Mission, who was in charge of the Catholic Mission Press. DeCruz also helped circulate this treatise among the Burmese under his influence. Likewise, *The Burman Herald*, *The Burman Messenger*, and the Sgau Karen paper (circa 1869) published the treatise gratis.[70] It is not clear if

68 1/1 (A) Accession 1083, 1867–68, File no. 5(2) "Treatise on Vaccination in the Vernacular" Box 1868 (1), Letter from the Deputy Commissioner of Tavoy to the Commissioner in Maulmain, dated 4 March 1868, NAUM, 55–56.

69 1/1 (A) Accession 1083, 1867–68, File no. 5(2) "Treatise on Vaccination in the Vernacular", Box 1868 (1), Letter from Charles Planck, Inspector General of Prisons, British Burma, to Horace Spearman, Esquire, Assistant Secretary to the Chief Commissioner, dated Rangoon, 2 April 1868, NAUM, 27.

70 *Report on Vaccination for 1868*, appendix, xiv–xv.

the treatise published in February 1869 was a modified version of Nisbet's original 1865 treatise, but it discussed the same themes. The "new" treatise devoted half its pages to explaining the difference between vaccination and variolation, focusing on the advantages of the former. This content obviously did not follow the suggestions made earlier by higher government officials.

Circumventing the government had its limitations. Nisbet complained that "none [of the newspapers] were distributed in the neighbourhood at public expense".[71] So, the treatise was circulated only among a very limited number of indigenous people and did not reach all whom Nisbet and the other civil surgeons desperately hoped to convince to accept vaccination.[72] He concluded that the entire effort was a failure and that it "merely serves to mark the interest taken in the subject by the responsible officer in charge".[73] In his view, government officers did not expect the treatise to have an effect on any of the adverse circumstances so long as variolation was still practised. His enthusiastic effort to circulate the treatise in the vernacular was ignored, or not appreciated, by the government. The only comment published on it was a negative assessment by Sanitary Commissioner Cowie. He wrote that he did not support the publication and circulation of the treatise because "I knew he could not afford the people the protection against Small Pox, he advised them to adopt in lieu of inoculation".[74] It is difficult to say how much influence Nisbet's treatise had on the civil surgeons who originally supported his plan. Government reports over a decade later, for example, refer to the civil medical officers in Prome having "prepared and circulated" a short account of vaccination, including its history and advantages.[75] We lack information, however, whether this treatise was based on Nisbet's or, indeed, if the officers merely forwarded the physician's original treatise itself. Nevertheless, in either case, Nisbet's hopes went unrealised in the short term, a consequence of the lack of government support and the independent course of action pursued by the medical officer.

71 Ibid.

72 *Report on Public Health and Statistics in British Burma for 1868*, 191–92.

73 *Report on Vaccination for 1868*, appendix, xiv–xv.

74 *Report on Public Health and Vital Statistics for 1869*, 48.

75 *RABB during 1880–81*, 126.

## *Conclusion*

Scholars have often viewed indigenous resistance to colonial vaccination in the context of anti-colonial nationalism, and in terms of the colonial violation of the indigenous body. Arnold, for example, argues that vaccination failed in British India in part because it became a symbol of colonialism and entered into the Indian nationalist discourse. Similarly, in Burma, village *wunthanu athins* (local nationalist organisations), connected to nationalist politicians in Rangoon, began to oppose vaccination as part of the overall struggle against colonialism in the 1920s. These organisations actively discouraged villagers from getting their children vaccinated. In the districts where *wunthanu athins* were most active, including Lower Chindwin, Meiktila, Sagaing, and Shwebo, there was a clear decline in the number of vaccinations and revaccinations, and they may also have contributed to the failure of the vaccination training school in Meiktila.[76] Nevertheless, indigenous resistance to vaccination and the preference for inoculation was not rooted in nationalism, for the nationalist discourse on vaccination never reached the levels seen in India and the issue in Burma was short-lived. Instead, the main factor affecting the indigenous acceptance of vaccination in Burma was the lack of communication between the colonial medical establishment and the Burmese population, especially indigenous doctors.

To convince the always evasive indigenous population to undergo vaccination, British medical officers turned to local officials for support, but these people frequently became yet another obstacle. Christian missionaries appeared to be promising agents to convince the Burmese of vaccination's blessings, but their influence was limited to the court elite in Upper Burma until 1885 and to ethnic minorities in Lower Burma into the twentieth century. To influence the Burmans who constituted a majority of Burma's population, some enthusiastic medical officers proposed launching their own propaganda by publishing and circulating treatises on vaccination in the vernacular. However, the lack of British government support nearly nullified this plan and, indeed, substantially limited its

[76] *RAB for 1922–1923*, 101; in the North-West Border Division during the year 1922–23, there was a decrease of 10,099 in the number of revaccinations. Ibid.

effect. Since the effort to "translate" vaccination to the indigenous population was half-hearted and inconsistent, it only made the Burmese more confused about the procedure's promised efficacy. As a result of the problems in developing a consistent propaganda programme, the colonial authorities abandoned efforts to pursue indigenous cooperation through propaganda and increasingly relied on legislation and the cultivation of indigenous agency (through enlisting Burmese vaccinators). It was thus not until the 1920s, after decades of legislation enforcing vaccination, that the colonial administration officially (as opposed to Nisbet's unofficial effort in the nineteenth century) undertook the promotion of vaccination in the popular print media. This occurred at a time when civil officers were more confident about the prospects of vaccination's success in the colony. In this way, propaganda came too late, because it followed rather than prompted the growing acceptance of vaccination among the indigenous population.

# 5

# *Inoculators*

In 1911, Major S. A. Harriss, the officiating Superintendent General of Vaccination in Burma, observed of the indigenous preference for inoculation, "The explosion of a bomb in a village would not be followed by a more deadly result than is brought about by the visit of an inoculator".[1] The prevailing historiography concerning the colonial discourse on inoculation, or variolation, characterised mainly by denigrating comments such as those of Harriss, tends to place it within a Eurocentric dichotomy: vaccination as the Western, superior prophylactic medicine versus inoculation as the non-Western, inferior, and dangerous practice. Inoculation is often associated with indigenous resistance to vaccination and considered the primary obstacle to its smooth progress. In the context of British India, the indigenous population's resistance to vaccination and preference for inoculation has often been examined with an emphasis on Indian culture and religion. Arnold offers the "raw secularity" theory in which he argues that Jennerian vaccination's lack of "ritual and dietary preparation", an important component of indigenous inoculation, made it an "irreligious" act, and therefore unpopular. He also suggests other reasons for the dislike of vaccination, one of them being the fear of polluting one's blood through arm-to-arm vaccination because the only indigenous subjects who agreed to become carriers of the virus belonged to the low castes or were untouchables.[2] Harish Naraindas argues that the primary reason variolation remained popular in India was because it was "part of therapeutics" while vaccination was "primarily prophylactic".[3]

1 *TRVB for 1908–09 to 1910–11*, 7.
2 Arnold, *Colonizing the Body,* 141–44.
3 Naraindas, "Care, Welfare, and Treason, 67–96.

Recent scholarship, however, has challenged this view. Niels Brimnes focuses on the ambiguous nature of this dichotomy in the case of the Madras Presidency where inoculation was unknown before the introduction of vaccination. He explains that the early colonial medical campaign against smallpox in Madras began with a rigorous promotion of inoculation, associating the technique with Europeans while attempting to "mask its indigenous roots" (in India). This colonial enthusiasm for inoculation, however, quickly died down with the introduction of Jennerian vaccination. With clear European origins, vaccination was promoted as safe and effective, though, in actuality, this was not the case. Colonial medical rhetoric now portrayed vaccination's competitor, inoculation, solely as an indigenous practice.[4] Brimnes thus makes the important point that the religio-cultural dichotomies were blurred and negotiated at different times at different places. Rather than focus on such blurred boundaries, Bhattacharya, Harrison, and Worboys pay close attention to the details of vaccination and inoculation operations and find that vaccinators in rural areas could obtain only "weak" lymph because of the inefficient transportation system. This inferior lymph forced them to alter their operation technique and make deeper incisions, leading to more painful vaccination operations. They further argue that the problems of post-vaccination complications in rural operations as well as the transmission of diseases such as syphilis through them made the procedure more dangerous and unreliable compared to variolation.[5]

Here, we examine variolation as a familiar mode of preventive medicine to the Burmese. Its operational technique played a role in encouraging indigenous preference for it by associating it with the Burmese "medical" custom of tattooing. Further, we look at the fluctuating and discordant policies and opinions among the colonial medical authorities on how to prohibit variolation. Last, we will show how Burmese inoculators were active agents of the colonial vaccination discourse. They not only enthusiastically convinced the indigenous population not to undergo vaccination, but also, more importantly, devised ways to circumvent the law and use the legal system against their dumfounded rulers.

[4] Niels Brimnes. "Variolation, Vaccination and Popular Resistance in Early Colonial South India," *Medical History* 48 (2004), 199–228.

[5] Bhattacharya, Harrison, and Worboys, *Fractured States*, 52–69.

## *Indigenous Inoculation*

Before the introduction of vaccination, inoculation had been established as the indigenous preventive medicine against smallpox in Burma, where it had had a presence since the end of the eighteenth century. According to Father Vicenzo Sangermano, a Catholic priest and medical practitioner in Burma in the late eighteenth century, Arakanese deportees to the Irrawaddy valley introduced inoculation to Burma after King Bodawhpaya's armies conquered the kingdom of Arakan in 1785. Arakan is in western Burma, on the eastern side of the Bay of Bengal, flanking the Indian subcontinent, with which it shares many things after centuries of cultural exchange.[6]

It should be stressed that any attempt to discuss inoculation as representing a set methodology would be fraught with problems. Robert Pringle's 1885 examination of inoculation in India, for example, described it as a single practice, whereas Bhattacharya, Harrison, and Worboys observe that this seeming uniformity masked an assortment of methodologies, albeit all based on the same basic principle (inducing resistance by introducing the human smallpox virus). In addition to individual differences, there were also broad regional differences, which is important to the present discussion. There was a general difference between inoculation operations in western India and southern India, on the one hand, and Bengal, on the other. In the former regions, smallpox lymph was introduced using lancets and razors, while in the latter, dried smallpox matter was introduced using a needle. Again, the differences in practices were not entirely uniform and there were variations within regions.[7] Nevertheless, the role of Arakan in the transmission of inoculation technology to Burma raises interesting questions about the kind of operation performed. Arakan's geographical position

[6] Atsuko Naono, "Inoculators, the Indigenous Obstacle to Vaccination in Colonial Burma", in *Medicine in Colonial Myanmar*, ed. Monique Skidmore (Copenhagen: NIAS), forthcoming; Vicenzo Sangermano, *Description of the Burmese Empire*, translated by William Tandy (Rome: Oriental Translation Fund of Great Britain and Ireland, 1833), 131.

[7] According to Bhattacharya, Harrison, and Worboys, in western and southern India, variolation was conducted with razors and lancets, but variolators in Bombay Presidency also operated with needles. Bhattacharya, Harrison, and Worboys, *Fractured States*, 53–55.

astride Bengal, the overlap of Bengali and Burmese cultures in Arakan, and the migration of Arakanese and Bengalis back and forth across their borders could help explain why Burmese inoculation technology in the nineteenth century shared important similarities with the method described in Bengal.

Unfortunately, for Burma, we do not have a nineteenth century example of the detailed kind Pringle provided of inoculation in India. Detailed British studies of inoculation in Burma do not appear until 1912. One reason for this was that the question whether inoculation was a viable alternative to vaccination was a moot point. Late nineteenth century and early twentieth century medical officers stationed in Burma came from a European context in which inoculation had already given way to vaccination. In their progressive view of medicine, inoculation represented a primitive stage in the development of prophylactic medicine. It was, in their eyes, no longer a valid competitor with vaccination, but yet another example of the "backward" state of indigenous medical practices that should be corrected. In 1908, for example, Entrican dismissed inoculation out of hand. He commented, "Inoculation has been given up by all except ignorant people, because it does more harm than good, and vaccination has been substituted for it".[8]

In the late nineteenth and twentieth centuries, a host of obstacles to the extension of vaccination in the subcontinent were listed in government reports, but in Burma, inoculation remained the main hurdle. The persistence and ubiquity of inoculation rivalry in Burma compared to its diminishing appeal elsewhere may thus have required focused attention. One officer who was intimately aware of the persistence of inoculation was Lieutenant-Colonel R. S. Castor (1862–1921), who served as the civil surgeon in Akyab in the mid-1890s and in Mandalay from the first decade of the twentieth century until he retired from the IMS in 1920. Castor was interested in the Burmese knowledge of diseases, as indicated by the publication of his *Nomenclature of Diseases in Burmese* in 1922. More importantly, in 1912, he attempted to share knowledge of Burmese inoculation practices with other colonial medical officers by publishing the first detailed British examination of this topic in the *Journal of Tropical Medicine and Hygiene*, justifying it on

[8] Entrican, *Notes for the Use of Vaccinators*, 26.

the fact that nothing had been published on vaccination in Burma in recent years.[9]

Castor provides the first serious and extensive description of the inoculation operation in Burma. Inoculators, he explains, were always male. According to him, the main tool used was the thorn. On occasion, the tattooist's needle was used, and, in a very small number of cases, glass from a broken bottle. All these served to make a single mark on each forearm, usually just above the wrist. Earlier colonial observations had been brief or ambiguous, usually only a sentence or two in reports on vaccination or public health. On the basis of this fragmentary evidence, it appears that in Burma, as in Bengal, dried smallpox scabs were used, sometimes mixed with milk. This matter was introduced by pricking the skin and inserting it into the opening with a thorn, needle, or piece of glass. A factor which may have helped to encourage the spread of this practice in Burma was that it required no major change in existing technologies, for skilled practitioners were already available to conduct operations in this manner. The Burmese tattooing operation was very similar to the inoculation method, with the tattooist using a sharp iron or bronze tool akin to a needle and applying pigment such as blue ink through a prick-by-prick motion.[10]

The basic principle involved in inoculation must have been easy to transfer to the Burmese spiritual context because tattooing was believed to deliver spiritual power to protect one from both mundane external forces such as gunshots, knife cuts or snake bites

[9] This article was based on an examination of 1,028 people (517 in Upper Burma, 393 in Lower Burma, and 118 in the Shan States) from 14 to 75 years of age (30 years on average), which found that 47 per cent of the Burmese in Upper Burma had been inoculated, 55 per cent in Lower Burma, and 15 per cent among the Shans. R. H. Castor, "Inoculation, Vaccination and Smallpox", *Journal of Tropical Medicine and Hygiene* 15, no.18 (1912), 278–81.

[10] Castor, "Inoculation, Vaccination and Smallpox", 278–81; Manning Nash, *The Golden Road to Modernity: Village Life in Contemporary Burma* (Chicago: University of Chicago Press, 1965), 180–81; Even though, in contrast to hill tribes, the custom of ornamental tattooing among lowland Burmese women was decreasing, the tattooers' art was still employed to add "a red beauty spot" on the female neck. Jordanna Bailkin, "Making Faces: Tattooed Women and Colonial Regimes", *History Workshop Journal* 59 (2005), 37.

and more harmful influences such as evil spirits.[11] Smallpox, as we know from several cases in nineteenth century Burma, was often viewed as a powerful, hostile spirit, and inoculation could easily have been presented as a means not unlike a tattoo that granted some kind of special protection against it. While we lack sufficient documentary evidence from the nineteenth century to support this contention with absolute certainty, it goes far in explaining the fact that many "indigenous medical practitioners" in Burma also practised tattooing. Finally, the custom of tattooing provided yet another reason for the successful spread of inoculation technology. The scale and duration of pain in tattooing was far greater than in inoculation, as was the risk of death. Burmese society made this ritual, which demanded enduring pain and bravely facing the risk of death, a test of manhood (although among some highland groups in Burma women were also tattooed, for different reasons) critical for securing a mate, for "a woman would have nothing to do with a man who did not exhibit the tattooed thigh".[12] Most Burmese would not have viewed the pain and risk involved in inoculation as major factors against it.

The role of the tattooist may indicate that inoculation was perceived by the people as "informal" medicine, outside the scope of the branches of "formal" Burmese medical practice. What formal Burmese medicine consisted of is open to debate, but a survey of available indigenous medical histories and the absence of inoculation in them provides some basis for the assertion that the practice of inoculation did not make one a *hsaya* (medical practitioner) though a *hsaya* may have practised inoculation during epidemics when all other remedies failed. According to the *Myanmar Taing-yin hse-pyinya Thamaing* ("History of Indigenous Medical Knowledge"), indigenous medical authorities made an effort to compile their knowledge so that it did not disappear, now that Burma had come under foreign rule. Such medical men were mostly Buddhist

[11] Max and Bertha Ferrars describe the tattooing operation, "Owing to the extent of surface involved, the process is most painful. It occupied days or weeks, according to the fortitude of the subject, who is drugged with opium for the occasion. The instrument has a handle weighted at the budd, and a long point of bronze, split like a ruling-pen". Max and Bertha Ferrars, *Burma* (Bangkok: Ava Publishing House, 1996), 13.

[12] Nash, *The Golden Road to Modernity*, 180–81.

monks who were well versed in medicine. For example, the head of the Buddhist order, Withoudathirasaha Thiyipawaya Dhammathenapati, composed a medical text that included Ayurvedic medicine as well as medical practices derived from Buddhist teachings such as the Winaya Pitala Mahawaga Vethinzahkanda. The most influential medical authorities emerged from the Taungtha medical group. The "great teacher", *hsaya* Hmoung (died 1877), composed a six-volume medical text and initiated most of what became known, and respected, as Taungtha medical knowledge. *Hsaya* Hmoung taught numerous important medical practitioners, including his own son U Ahsaya (who was also a prominent Buddhist monk at Taungtha), *hsaya* Hme, U Kyantha, U Phomin, and *hsaya* Ke. After Hmoung's death, his Taungtha medical knowledge survived through the British period, all the way to the present. To preserve indigenous medical knowledge, numerous Buddhist monks compiled and composed medical treatments in the tradition of Hmoung. *Hsaya* Hme, one of Hmoung's pupils, composed a medical text entitled *Kyauloungnika* after repeated requests by two other Buddhist monks, U Sanda and U Zayaga, both from Thandwe district.

Among the many medical texts on indigenous medicine produced by practitioners of the Taungtha school of indigenous medicine, there were numerous texts that prescribed treatments for smallpox other than inoculation. In 1894, one of Hmoung's pupils, the "great layman", U Pantha, composed a medical treatise on smallpox called *Byamiwithara*, based on his own experiences and the traditions of Dat treatment. This text became a favourite among medical practitioners for the treatment of smallpox. Besides Pantha, U Kyantha, another graduate of the Taungtha school, composed a medical text called *Paramyithalekhanya Taungtha Kyaungloungnika apye kyan*. In it, he explained the treatment of smallpox, its symptoms, stages, and characteristics while laying down what a patient should eat and drink. This text has become an indigenous classic for the treatment of smallpox by Burmese medical *hsayas*.[13] It is clear that such indigenous medical men, many of them respected Buddhist monks, played an important role in fostering indigenous medical knowledge regarding smallpox and circulated this

[13] *Myanma Taing-yin hse-pinya Thamaing* [History of Indigenous Medical Knowledge] (Yangon: Department of Ministry of Health, 1978), 103–4.

knowledge through medical texts. However, none of the indigenous medical texts examined by the author described inoculation procedures per se.

## *Problems with Translation*

Vernacular public notices were one of a small range of print media through which the colonial medical authorities sought to directly communicate with the indigenous population on medical matters. Nevertheless, they seem to have been of no help in clarifying the difference between vaccination and inoculation. Whatever colonial expectations were, this was no simple task. Translating into the vernacular involved problem of finding a vocabulary that carried the same meaning and experience as the original. Alton Becker argues that the obstacles of "exuberance" and "deficiency" complicate the translator's task. At the moment of translation, a translated word may be "exuberant" because it says more than what was meant in the original, or "deficient" because it may convey less than what was desired in the original. The translator seeks to escape the lack of direct equivalents in language by an interpretive process that digs deep into the contextual realm.[14]

Bilingual government publications were a constant source of confusion due to the need for strict legalese in both English and Burmese. The Rangoon municipality published on 11 April 1902 revised bye-laws on the registration of births and deaths under section 142, clause (c), of the Burma Municipal Act of 1898. These bye-laws gave the health officer superintending authority over the register of births and deaths in Rangoon. Instructions for the birth certificate stated, in English, "You are hereby informed that unless your child is vaccinated successfully within the period of 6 months from this date, legal proceedings will be taken against you under the provisions of the Vaccination Act".[15] For a British or Indian health officer, this was a straightforward statement, lacking nuance. For most Burmese, however, a reading of the vernacular text of the same statement was ambiguous, for it used *kyauk htou gyin* (smallpox

[14] A. L. Becker, ed., *Writing on the Tongue* (Ann Arbor: University of Michigan Centers for South and Southeast Asian Studies, 1989), 1–10.

[15] *Rangoon Municipality Handbook*, sixth edition (Rangoon: Superintendent of Government Printing, Burma. 1908), 240–42.

vaccination) for vaccination and not *nwa-kyauk htou gyin* (cowpox vaccination). The Burmese translation of "inoculation" was also *kyauk htou gyin*. Various vernacular terms used for vaccination and inoculation in the government print media would thus have caused considerable confusion among the indigenous population about the operation their children had to undergo.[16]

As for the translation of "vaccination" and "inoculation" into the Burmese *kyauk htou gyin*, the translator, who was most likely Burmese, may have viewed "vaccination" as merely a slightly modified method of "inoculation", which the indigenous population was familiar with and understood. Their cognitive realm would not have registered "vaccination" as substantially different from indigenous "inoculation". Therefore, there was no reason to develop a new vernacular term for "vaccination". It can also be asserted that even today in the West and other regions of the world, the words inoculation, vaccination and immunisation are treated as if they were synonyms and often used interchangeably, applicable equally to smallpox and other diseases. However, to explain the desperation found in the reports of the colonial Vaccination Department to clarify the difference between vaccination and inoculation, more attention has to be paid to the ways in which these two words were treated in vernacular translation. The indigenous translator would

[16] Colonial Burma was not alone in the conflict over the terminological distinction between inoculation and vaccination. This was partly due to a lack of direction and methods to "keep up" with the vicissitudes of the integration of Western and indigenous medical technologies into a single body of medical knowledge. In Japan, smallpox inoculation and cowpox vaccination were both referred to as *syutou*. Before cowpox vaccination was successfully introduced in Japan in 1849 in Nagasaki, the term *syutou* was used to describe smallpox inoculation. However, after its introduction, cowpox vaccination was also widely called *syutou* and vaccination stations were officially termed *syutou-sho*. For example, Ogata Syunsaku of Akizuki-han published the first textbook on smallpox inoculation as *Syutouu hissu-ben* in 1795. Fujii Naohisa, "Meiji-zen Honpo Sippei-shi", in *Meiji-zen Nihon Igaku-shi* (Tokyo: Nihon gakujyutu shinko-kai, 1955), 2: 308. *Otamagaike syutou-sho* which was established in 1858 is the origin of the medical department of the Tokyo University. *Tokyo daigaku igaku-bu hyakunen-shi* (Tokyo: Tokyo daigaku shuppan-kaim, 1967), 4–5. Further, while both smallpox inoculation and cowpox vaccination were available in Japan, both methods were called *syutou* until the Meiji period when *syutou* came to mean only vaccination.

not have been working in isolation, for many of the British among the Vaccination Department staff also understood Burmese and should have been able to catch the incongruity between the Burmese translation and the English original, had they paid close attention. So, despite the colonial government's concern over the confusion between vaccination and inoculation, the ambiguity was probably also due in part to inadequate colonial concern for, or ignorance of, the nuances of the Burmese language, for a clear distinction was available in vernacular medical texts of the period. To take one example, *hsaya* Htout's *Ingalei-hseì-kyan* translated vaccination as *nwa-kyauk htou nyi*.[17] In *nwa-kyauk htou nyi*, *nwa* means cow and *kyauk* means pox or smallpox, *htou* means to poke or jab, and *nyi* means method. Without *nwa*, *kyauk htou gyin* could mean either vaccination or inoculation.

A similar terminological problem occurred in the case of rinderpest. A report by G. E. Evans, the Superintendent of the Civil Veterinary Department, in 1900 suggested that the negative indigenous view of vaccination even filtered down to Burmese cattle owners in rural areas. Among this group, the terms *kyauk-pauk* or *kyauk-yawga*, which were used for human smallpox, were also commonly used to refer to rinderpest. When veterinary officers visited villages to inoculate cattle for rinderpest, they used the term *kyauk-hto* or inoculation (for smallpox), because they believed that indigenous owners would be more cooperative given the popularity of inoculation. However, to the Burmese, *kyauk-hto* also meant vaccination. Using the term "vaccinate", veterinary officers found, had "the effect of making some owners shy". Ultimately, the Veterinary Department dropped the terms connected with vaccination altogether, creating instead a new term, *ahlun-kaungthau-se*, or "very good medicine".[18]

In the early twentieth century, the colonial medical authorities in Burma paid closer attention to the issue of communicating medical concepts with greater accuracy. In the Burmese translation of *Notes for the Use of Vaccinators*, written by Entrican, vaccination was again ambiguously translated as *kyauk htou hnan gyin* in the

[17] Hsaya Htout, *Ingalei-hseì-kyan* (Rangoon: Bengalee Job Printing Press, 1881), 138.

[18] IOR/V/24/4409, V.2., 1891–92 to 1907–08, Annual Report of the Civil Veterinary Department, Burma for the year ending 31 March 1900.

title. However, in the text, the Burmese translation added certain words to distinguish clearly between vaccination and inoculation. Vaccination and inoculation were translated as *nwa-kyauk htou hnan gyin* ("cowpox vaccination" or "poking") and *myanma kyauk htou hnan gyin* ("myanma smallpox inoculation" or "poking") respectively. Although not intended for the general population, this translation would have been used by Burmese vaccinators, so some progress had definitely been made. This distinction was further emphasised by the addition of "Myanma" (Burmese) to inoculation to stress its indigeneity even though the English original simply said "inoculation".[19] Therefore, a clear distinction between inoculation and vaccination was available and could have been used if one chose to, as did the translator of Entrican's text.

## *Inoculation as the Enemy*

A careful examination of the colonial medical discourse on inoculation in nineteenth century Burma reveals a great diversity of opinion on the practice of inoculation. Some civil surgeons accepted that inoculation was a viable alternative to vaccination while others saw it as a necessary evil that had to be tolerated until the vaccination establishment had the ability to protect the entire population. Most, however, vehemently opposed it because it was a major cause, alongside ineffective lymph, for the delay in popularising vaccination. From the beginning of vaccination operations in the mid-1860s to the late 1920s, colonial medical officers repeatedly reported the Burmese preference for inoculation as a factor that retarded the progress of vaccination operations.[20]

Underlying the colonial medical establishment's concerns over inoculation was a different understanding of medicine. Although mainstream indigenous medical practitioners may not have considered inoculation to fall within the sphere of proper medicine, they appear to have voiced little opposition to it. Burmese medical customs allowed for heterogeneous solutions to medical complaints, and if one specialist in a particular field of indigenous medicine failed, there was little resentment on the part of the

19 *Kyauk htou hsaya mya thin kya le la yan, kyauk hto hnan gyin hnin kyanma gyin saing ya hma su mya*. Entrican, *Notes for the Use of Vaccinations*, 26, 31.

20 *RABB during 1866–67*, 31.

practitioner if the patient turned to a specialist in another field for help. As early colonial doctors, such as MacDonald in Prome, found, there was simply no single system of Burmese medicine. This was in sharp contrast to the spirit of colonial medicine which promoted a monolithic "scientific medicine", discouraging those that it failed from pursuing alternative cures.

Colonial doctors attributed a number of dangers to inoculation, such as it serving as a major conduit for the spread of smallpox. It is interesting to pay close attention to the words and phrases used by them in their reports, alluding to the mysterious nature of the outbreaks and also using the opportunity to cast aspersions on inoculation. MacDonald pointed to inoculation as the "principal cause" of a smallpox epidemic that broke out in his district in January 1867 though the only reason for this was "the mildness of the epidemic and its slow spreading tendency".[21] Parker, the civil surgeon in Toungoo, demonstrated a determination to blame inoculation despite having little proof for doing so, "Inoculation is very commonly practised here, and often, as of course must be the case, gives the patient a severe attack of the disease it is meant to ward off".[22] Vinton, who had vaccinated many Karens and Shans over the years, had become such a supporter of the anti-inoculation cause that he blamed inoculation for introducing smallpox "where it had not existed previously".[23] The civil surgeon in Mergui, Donnelly, claimed in a report, again without offering any clear evidence, that smallpox was spread in Burma more often by inoculation than by any other means.[24] The deputy commissioner in Tavoy thus explained the practice of inoculation in a letter to the commissioner in Maulmain in 1868,

> Inoculation is practised here only when warning is received of the approach of the disease from neighbouring Districts, and is not practised at other times as it is said not to be then effectual and its tendency to spread the disease, is always feared.[25]

21 *RPHVS for 1867*, 15, appendix I, 47.
22 *RVB for 1867–68*, 42.
23 *RVB for 1871–72*, 9.
24 *RPHVS for 1869*, 139.
25 NAUM 1/1 (A) Accession 1083, 1867–1868, 5 (2) "Treatises on Vaccination in the Vernacular" (1868/1), Letter from the Deputy Commissioner of Tavoy to the Commissioner at Maulmain, dated 4 March 1868, 55.

Colonial civil surgeons were aware of dissenting voices among the indigenous population, but ignored them. MacDonald interviewed "several Burmese of respectability" and jotted down what they knew about inoculation. He was told that it was "a perfectly safe and justifiable operation" because "they never saw a single casualty resulting from inoculation". Further, these Burmese described the mildness of smallpox when it developed in the inoculated. The symptoms were only "slight feverishness", "a rash on the body and arm", or pits on the face which "rapidly disappear".[26] One of the indigenous *hsayas* confirmed the safety of the practice by telling MacDonald that he had seen only 12 deaths occur because of inoculation.[27] Special reasons were cited to explain why inoculation had been unsuccessful in some cases. When Daniel Henry Cullimore discussed inoculation operations in 1885, "intelligent natives" told him "a second inoculation is occasionally necessary".[28] He was also told some indigenous people were "not susceptible to various inoculations" because of "the hereditary influence of the disease or some occult causes".[29] Convictions such as this led to a general belief among the Burmese that vaccination was "an inferior method of protection to inoculation".[30] To nineteenth-century colonial doctors, these views were very unsound.

The colonial argument against inoculation failed to convince the indigenous population because it was too extreme; the problems of inoculation were not quite as sweeping as the civil surgeons argued. Gradually, however, a perhaps more enlightened generation of colonial doctors in Burma began to take the indigenous argument seriously. They did not accept that inoculation was as effective as vaccination but were more willing to understand why the Burmese believed so. In the late 1910s, for example, Entrican provided a more favourable view of Burmese inoculation.

> Apart from its being a time honoured practice, I believe the chief cause of its popularity is the absence in the majority of cases of any troublesome symptoms, such as sometimes follow vaccination under insanitary

[26] *RVB for 1867–68*, 35–36.

[27] MacDonald, *The Practice of Medicine Among the Burmese*, 48, footnote.

[28] Edward Balfour, *The Cyclopaedia of India and of Eastern and Southern Asia*, 3rd ed. (London: Bernard Quaritch, 1885), 3: 983.

[29] Balfour, *Cyclopaedia*, 3: 983–84.

[30] *RVB for 1867–68*, 35.

> conditions. The inoculated child may of course develop generalised small-pox and die, this risk is clearly recognised, but accepted, because in the majority of cases the after-effects are almost nil. A small pock with perhaps 2 or 3 still smaller ones round it, is the usual course of an inoculation, and the children require little if any attention.[31]

Entrican thus admitted that at a personal level inoculation may have been justifiably viewed as a much safer operation than vaccination in Burma. His observation reflected an awareness of why the indigenous population believed that inoculation was safe, or at least presented more advantages than disadvantages. His comment, however, did not amount to a major change in his general view that vaccination was superior to inoculation. He still maintained, for instance, that inoculation was the "folly of ignorant people". He also suspected inoculation was to blame in some smallpox epidemics, for he further said, "That the inoculated child may spread infection and give rise to a severe epidemic of small-pox, is either not recognised, or else considered outside the sphere of human action and fittingly left in the hands of Providence".[32] Nevertheless, Entrican appears to have been more willing than many of his predecessors and peers to understand that inoculation was not a monolithic evil.

## *Legislation*

Colonial medical authorities noticed a clear division in the smallpox prevention landscape when it came to the vaccination versus inoculation issue. This divide ran between urban (municipal) dwellers and rural (non-municipal) dwellers. In urban areas, medical officers could exercise their authority to ensure vaccination was adopted. In addition, a more reliable transportation system connected the major towns and this made fresh and more effective lymph available to urban dwellers. This, in turn, made vaccination operations in these areas more successful than in the countryside. The rural areas were outside municipal limits, making it difficult for medical officers to intervene in local behaviour on a regular basis. This also meant the government could not keep a close eye on indigenous medical practitioners who carried out inoculations

31 *TRVB for 1917–18 to 1919–20*, 7.

32 Ibid.

outside the towns. The problem of not being able to reach people in the remote interior to demonstrate the efficacy of vaccination contributed to the government's frustration over the tenaciousness of inoculation. Superintendent General of Vaccination Williams reported in late 1908,

> Inoculation is still practised freely in non-municipal areas. In the absence of facilities for obtaining the services of vaccinators, and also by the reason of their distrust in the efficacy of vaccination, as a protection against small-pox, the rural population continues to resort to inoculation whenever they are threatened by an epidemic of small-pox.[33]

As early as the late 1860s, the colonial medical establishment in Burma had considered ways to actively oppose inoculation though they lacked a firm legal basis to do so. Many medical officers urged the authorities to take some action to control inoculation if prohibition was not an option.[34] Some even manipulated existing legislation to force inoculators to cease their operations. The deputy commissioner in Shwegyeen threatened inoculators "under a section of the Penal Code against spreading the 'contagious and infectious disease'".[35] Although the existing laws were thus used by the colonial medical authorities, the absence of legislation specifically targeted at inoculation made this a difficult task. Civil surgeons and other British authorities in Burma passionately debated whether the colonial government should take the step of making the practice of inoculation illegal. One of the most vocal proponents of anti-inoculation legislation was civil surgeon Cowie, who was frustrated by the stagnant state of the vaccination campaign and the opportunities that had been missed to reverse the situation. He lamented, "Herewith we had [lost] a chance of preventing the continuance of Small Pox into the months most favorable to its propagation, by prohibiting the inoculators extending their filthy and dangerous practice."[36] But there was a vocal minority who argued that the time was not ripe to make inoculation illegal. For example, Lieutenant-Colonel Ryan asked in 1870,

> Would it be right then to rob people of a safeguard of this kind [inoculation] by making its adoption a criminal offence against the State

33 *TRVB for 1905–06 to 1907–08*, 3.
34 *RVB for 1871–72*, 8–9.
35 *RPHVS for 1869*, 49.
36 Ibid.

simply because we have hitherto failed to convince them that vaccination is a safer means to the same end than that the benefits of which have been proved to their satisfaction over and over again?[37]

Nevertheless, the views of this minority were drowned out by the majority that was concerned vaccination was losing its battle for the hearts and minds of the Burmese. Cowie complained about the same time as Ryan's sympathetic plea that poor handling of the situation by medical staff during the years of trial and error in the 1860s had weakened the case for vaccination.

It will take a long time, and require great care and supervision in the management of the practice [of vaccination] to restore it to the position in which I left it in [Prome in] 1862, when all classes not only believed in it, but were eager to receive its benefits.[38]

It would be another decade before special anti-inoculation legislation became available. It was then produced in Calcutta to resist inoculation in greater India, not specifically to deal with the problem in Burma. The Government of India attempted to ban inoculation through the enactment of the Vaccination Act (XIII, of 1880) that prohibited inoculation under section 6.

In any local area to which the provisions of this Act apply, inoculation shall be prohibited; and no person who has undergone inoculation shall enter such area before the lapse of forty days from the date of the operation, without a certificate from a medical practitioner, of such class as the Local Government may from time to time by written order authorise to grant such certificates, stating that such person is no longer likely to produce small-pox by contact or near approach.[39]

This Act also gave local colonial officers the authority to punish those who violated it with sentences of up to three months in prison, a 200 rupee fine, or both.[40] The Act, however, applied only to specified municipalities and cantonments. In Burma, it did not go as far as local medical officers wished, for here the main concern was with inoculation in the hinterland.

The difficulties of using the Act to prohibit inoculation in rural Burma were demonstrated in several prominent court cases in the

37 *Report on Vaccination for 1868*, 24.

38 *RPHVS for 1869*, appendix, ix.

39 Government of India, *The Burma Code*, 88.

40 Ibid., 92.

late nineteenth century. This left colonial medical officers at a loss about how they could actually use it to combat the indigenous practice. In one such case, a Burmese practitioner named Nga San Pu inoculated some children in 1899 in the village of Kyithe in Prome district. The local civil surgeon dutifully reported what he believed to be an operation that was illegal under the terms of the Act to the deputy commissioner of Prome. The case was passed on to the sub-divisional officer in Shwedaung, for the village was under his jurisdiction, the deputy commissioner asking him to treat the case under the Indian Penal Code (section 269 and section 299–109). The sub-divisional officer then transferred the case to the *myo-ouk*, Maung Lu Gale, who was also the second-class magistrate in Shwedaung. As all the colonial officers in this chain had apparently hoped, Nga San Pu was found guilty as charged. He was sentenced to either a fine (five rupees) or imprisonment (four days). The four Burmese parents whose children had been inoculated received slightly less severe sentences, the fine being set at four rupees or imprisonment (also for four days). When the dust settled, however, the district magistrate in Prome was unhappy that the sentences had not been more severe. He sent the case for review to the judicial commissioner, Lower Burma, complaining that the inoculation, which had caused an outbreak of smallpox in the village, deserved a harsher sentence. Ultimately, the judgement was thrown out altogether, not because it was not harsh enough but because the colonial officers did not understand the proper procedures for making the Act applicable to specific cases.

More important than the procedural mistakes made by the colonial officers in the Nga San Pu case was their misunderstanding of the legal status of inoculation in terms of the 1880 Act. As Judicial Commissioner A. R. Birks explained, though section 6 of the Act prohibited inoculation in specified areas, it did not go so far as making inoculation illegal per se. As Kyithe village was outside such specified areas, Nga San Pu had not committed an offence under the Act. Birks suggested that the colonial officers forget about the 1880 Act in the present case and pursue prosecution under a different law. Since inoculation might be dangerous, he recommended that the district magistrate consider declaring the practice of inoculation in a non-municipal area under his jurisdiction to be against the interests of public health, under section 133 of the Criminal Procedure Code.

If such an order was issued, its violation would be punishable under section 188 of the Indian Penal Code, so long as the inoculators were given a reasonable opportunity to present their case on the safety of the operation. Birks ruled,

> It may be necessary in the interest of the public to prohibit the practice outside of the areas referred to in the Act. In that case the District Magistrate should draw up a proceeding, and after taking the evidence of the Civil Surgeon on the point he can issue orders to be served personally on the inoculators under section 133, Criminal Procedure Code, to show cause why the practice of their trade should not be suppressed as being injurious to the health of the community. If sufficient cause is not shown the order can be made absolute and its violation would be punishable under section 188, Penal Code. The sentences now passed [against the inoculator and the Burmese parents] are illegal. The convictions are set aside and the fines if paid will be refunded.[41]

The complicated procedures, special circumstances, and large amount of paperwork required for prosecuting just one inoculator was a far cry from the simple legal remedy for which civil surgeons in Burma had hoped. Nor did matters improve much in the remaining years of the century. In 1900, for example, virtually the same judgement was delivered when another district magistrate's condemnation of an inoculation operation was overturned. In this case, three Burmese were tried for practising inoculation, alleged to be an offence under section 269 of the Indian Penal Code. Again, since section 269 did not, in the higher court's opinion, make inoculation punishable per se, it was up to the prosecution to demonstrate that the three Burmese conducted inoculation "if not unlawfully, at least negligently". The judge in this case stated,

> This is the difficult word in the section. It must have some meaning. The section cannot be read as if the words unlawfully or negligently were omitted. Yet, except by omitting these words, it is difficult to see how the deliberate practice of inoculation by a person qualified to perform it where no negligence in the performance of the operation is alleged, can be held to be punishable under the section.[42]

41 *A Reprint of the Printed Judgments of the Court of the Judicial Commissioner, Lower Burma, and the Special Court for the Period extended from 1893–1900* (Rangoon: Superintendent, Government Printing, 1902), 546.

42 Penal Code-269. *The Upper Burma Rulings, 1897–1901: Criminal* (Rangoon: Superintendent, Government Printing and Stationery, Burma, 1931), 1: 280.

Burmese inoculators had also learnt how to actively use the colonial legal system to their advantage. In one case, when a township officer convicted an indigenous inoculator for an "illegal" operation, he successfully appealed to the Chief Court and had the lower court's judgement overturned. The inoculator then practised his trade freely in his area, carrying with him the written judgement of the Chief Court as proof that he had been granted permission to perform inoculation legally. This was just one of several such cases reported by the civil surgeons.

The new "certificate" system for vaccination also backfired on the British. As argued elsewhere,[43] in an effort to convert indigenous inoculators into government vaccinators, the government awarded "certificates of competency" to those who switched sides. The certificates were prized by the inoculators turned vaccinators, but often not for the reasons intended. To the dismay of the Vaccination Department, British civil surgeons discovered cases where the new vaccinators, certificates in hand, not only performed vaccinations incorrectly, but also continued to provide inoculations under the guise of vaccination. In Pegu, the civil surgeon complained that inoculators were practising openly with the vaccinator's "certificate" as proof of their authority and that they also carried copies of the Chief Court's order stating that inoculation was not illegal. Due to such incidents, the Vaccination Department began to grow suspicious of the motives of inoculators seeking certification. It was also worried that such certificates would give vaccination a bad name if a smallpox outbreak was caused by inoculations masquerading as vaccination.

The Vaccination Department moved to end the system of granting certificates in 1902, when its superintendent formally prohibited the issue of such documents in Burma. Though applications by indigenous *hsayas* for vaccinator training, and thus status, came to a halt in Rangoon, the municipality's shortage of medical staff meant that there remained other opportunities for circumventing the restrictions on the practice of inoculation. One such avenue was provided by the permitted category of "private vaccinator". Under this system, the municipality allowed indigenous *hsayas* to conduct vaccinations on their own, without the supervision of the Rangoon

[43] Naono, "Inoculators, the Indigenous Obstacle to Vaccination in Colonial Burma", 4.

Health Department. The municipality simply provided the lymph to these vaccinators. Sanitary Commissioner Williams praised the motives of the Rangoon municipal committee because he believed that they were not only philanthropic, but also "humane", the Burmese being more willing to accept vaccination from indigenous operators. Nevertheless, he also criticised this system because it hampered the work of the Vaccination Department in that the private vaccinators could charge "considerable fees from their patients", which exceeded the salary of municipal vaccinators, thus reducing the attractiveness of being employed by the government. Even worse, this system again made it possible for them to carry out inoculations with what appeared to be government sanction. The civil surgeons, he explained, considered that "such private vaccinators do little real vaccination work, and that many of them practice inoculation".[44]

William's decision to ban the distribution of lymph to private practitioners drew a hostile response from the Rangoon municipal committee, which resented provincial interference in its affairs. M. Laurie, the president of the committee, immediately sought to demonstrate the regularity of the municipality's practice by writing to his counterparts in Madras, Bombay and Calcutta, asking for reports on their policies to do witn private vaccinators. Though these three municipalities reported that they distributed vaccine lymph to private vaccinators, two of them, Bombay and Madras, did so only to demonstrably qualified individuals. The Lieutenant-Governor of Burma therefore agreed with William's decision to prohibit the distribution of lymph to private vaccinators and rejected the municipal committee's request that this injunction be set aside.[45]

[44] IOR/P/7791, File. No. 2Z-5, Pt. I, No. 1124–2Z–5, from D. Shearme, Esq., ICS, Secretary to the Government of Burma, to the Sanitary Commissioner, Burma, dated 25 March 1908; IOR/P/7791, File. No. 2Z-5, Pt. I, No. 2469–2 V. R., from Major C.E. Williams, MD, DPH, IMS, Sanitary Commissioner, Burma, to the Secretary to the Government of Burma, dated 11 April 1908.

[45] IOR/P/7791, File. No. 2Z-5, Pt. II, No. 571-4P-3, from M. Laurie, Esq., MVO, ICS, President, Rangoon Municipal Committee, to the Secretary to the Government of Burma, dated 3 July 1908; IOR/P/7791, File. No. 2Z-5, Pt. II, No. 306-2Z-5, from D. Shearme, Esq., ICS, Secretary to the Government of Burma, to the President, Rangoon Municipal Committee, dated 8 August 1908.

Over the half century between the 1860s and the early 1900s, relatively few Burmese inoculators were successfully prosecuted under the available laws. Colonial medical authorities had hoped that general Indian legislation would give them the legal means they needed to combat inoculation, but frequently found that the legal system, if not the legislation, helped protect the inoculators more than it punished them. In the next few years, however, legislation designed to specifically address the competition between vaccination and inoculation in Burma would emerge. The new legislation for which the Vaccination Department had hoped was produced in the chambers of the Lt. Governor's legislative council, an advisory body that proposed legislation the Lt. Governor could approve or reject. The members of this body represented the colonial elite. In other words, it comprised some prominent Europeans, a small sampling of wealthy Indian and Chinese merchants, and one or two Western-educated Burmese professionals, all of whom were sympathetic to causes that favoured colonial rule. On 29 August 1908, one of the more outspoken councilmen, Walter Francis Rice, brought a Bill to the legislative council which proposed prohibiting inoculation in local areas. His aim was to gradually extend the prohibition of inoculation to rural areas, where indigenous inoculators were most active and where the Vaccination Act was not applicable, and get more people in these areas to take to vaccination. The Bill was referred to a select committee comprising Charles Philip Radford-Young, F. C. Gates and Maung Ket, an anglophile. A few weeks later, in September 1908, Rice presented the select committee's report on the Bill to the legislative council, announcing that since no amendments had been recommended by the public, the committee did not think it necessary to change the Bill in any way. The Bill was then approved.[46]

It remains uncertain who Rice or the select committee meant when they referred to the "public" and how public opinion was solicited. Less than a month had passed between the time the Bill was proposed and it being passed into an Act, which afforded little time for the publication of official notifications, much less their translation into Burmese, if indeed any such effort was made. The details of the August 29 council meeting and the Bill were

[46] "Burma Legislative Council", *Rangoon Times* (Saturday, 29 August 1908), 11.

published in the English-language press, such as the *Rangoon Times*, but this could hardly have reached the general Burmese population, nor was there enough time to allow the Burmese to debate, in a meaningful fashion, how desirable the Bill was. It is probable that most Burmese, aside from the Westernised, English-speaking elite in Rangoon, did not learn of the Bill until well after it had become an Act, much too late for them to express an opinion about it if they wanted to.[47]

Apparently, the Burma Prohibition of Inoculation and Licensing of Vaccinators Act, 1908, was not successful in altering the local preference for inoculation. Indigenous inoculators again found ways to circumvent the restrictions imposed by it and, in 1915, a Bill was introduced in the legislative council to amend it. It was now argued that smallpox was caused by methods "not falling strictly within the meaning of the term 'inoculation' as defined in clause (5) of section 2 of the Vaccination Act, 1880".[48] This clause defined "inoculation" as any operation performed with the object of producing the disease of smallpox in any person by means of variolous matter. The methods at issue now included "the feeding of children with small-pox scabs mixed with jaggery, and the snuffing of pounded small-pox scabs into the nostrils".[49] These procedures were not strictly considered to be "operations", which was an essential part of the definition of "inoculation" in the 1908 Act.

The indigenous means of evading legislative restrictions, such as those that emerged in 1915, indicate that inoculators were attempting to escape the "controlled conditions" established to sustain British colonial rule in Burma. According to nineteenth-century British reports, indigenous inoculation was an operation which included inserting dried smallpox scabs mixed with milk into the body of the patient. No reports of the snuffing method or of feeding patients a mixture of jaggery and smallpox scabs were heard of in Burma before 1915. So, it is probably the case that some

[47] Ibid.

[48] "Abstract of the Proceedings of the Council of the Lieutenant-Governor of Burma" (1915), 403.

[49] Ibid; The Vaccination Act, 1880. Act No. XIII of 1880, in *The Burma Hand-book of Rural Self Government: Act and Rules,* Parts I and II (Rangoon: Superintendent, Government Printing and Stationery, Union of Burma), 1: 136.

indigenous inoculators studied the technical details of the term "inoculation" in the Act and changed their method, allowing them to continue their trade and evade criminal prosecution. Frederic Cooper and Ann Laura Stoler, in examining the issue of colonies being sites of European exploitation, have argued,

> What Europeans encountered in the colonies was not open terrain for economic domination, but people capable of circumventing and undermining the principles and practices on which extraction or capitalist development was based.[50]

Burmese inoculators reacted to colonial legislation in a similar way. They were not simply passive recipients of colonial regulations but active participants who sought out new ways to "circumvent and undermine" legislative obstacles to their advantage.

## *Conclusion*

Colonial medical authorities saw inoculators as serious obstacles in the way of getting the indigenous population to accept vaccination. First, the Burmese preference for inoculation was often viewed as an unavoidable consequence of the lack of effective lymph until around the beginning of the twentieth century. Second, when fresh lymph was unavailable or post-vaccination treatment was inappropriate, vaccination caused serious complications and children sometimes contracted other maladies such as typhoid. Indigenous inoculation seems to have rarely had such side effects. Third, vaccination, which involved making a couple of painful insertions with a lancet, was more painful than inoculation, which involved only a puncturing of the skin. Fourth, vaccination, unlike inoculation, did not provide life-long immunity with a single operation and Burmese parents did not like submitting their children to numerous revaccinations. Such disadvantages may have contributed to developing the way the Burmese perceived vaccination. The indigenous population did not view vaccination as a "safer" or "superior" prophylactic. Rather, it viewed it as "inferior" to indigenous inoculation. This belief was the result

50 Frederic Cooper and Ann Laura Stoler, eds., *Tensions of Empire: Colonial Cultures in a Bourgeois World* (Berkeley: University of California Press, 1997), 5.

of several factors. First, the distinction between inoculation and vaccination had not been made clear to the indigenous population. We know that the Burmese did not often know which operation they were submitting to. This was partly because of indigenous inoculators who pretended to be vaccinators while carrying out inoculations. These ambiguous agents confounded a public already confused by the lack of colonial attention to subtle differences in translation. In addition, the indigenous population probably found it easier to resort to inoculators because their techniques and equipment were already a ubiquitous part of the local landscape. The same could be said of the inoculators themselves, who, in their various roles as tattooists or native medical practitioners were familiar to the people in the areas where they practised. Without a similar local presence in much of the colony, especially outside the major towns, the colonial medical authorities found competing with inoculators difficult, if not impossible, in many areas. This encouraged the vaccination establishment to pursue legislation to bring inoculators to heel. But such legislation was frequently ineffective with indigenous inoculators finding ways to either circumvent the law or use it in their favour, undermining the relevance of what the authorities saw as a powerful control mechanism. Ultimately, colonial efforts to suppress inoculation in Burma had little success until the late 1920s.

# 6

# *Vaccinators*

Success in overcoming the technical impediments to vaccination did not bring the Vaccination Department much closer to extending vaccination in Burma. Crucially, it still failed to elicit the cooperation of the indigenous population. This was partly because it failed to control the Burmese inoculators. From the start, the Vaccination Department used non-European vaccinators in Burma to support its civil surgeons. In the years that followed, when colonial vaccination efforts began to cover the indigenous population as well as foreigners, indigenisation of the vaccination staff was viewed as a necessary, and hopefully inexpensive, means of obtaining greater cooperation from the people.

Winning popular support was a temporary stage in the vaccination programme. Colonial doctors tried and failed to popularise vaccination among the Burmese, an effort which led them to view the people almost as a troublesome enemy. We will examine how the colonial government attempted to make vaccination operations effective in Burma by focusing on the complex ways in which its relations with the indigenous vaccinators developed. We will also investigate how the medical establishment prepared the ground for educating indigenous vaccinators as well as the general population about vaccination. This involves tackling many questions. Is it valid, for example, to view the Vaccination Department in colonial Burma as a monolithic force that exercised its authority evenly throughout the colony? Why did the British choose some Burmese as potential collaborators and how did they seek to cultivate such collaboration? Who was defined by the medical establishment as "Burmese" and why? The answers to these questions help to explain why the colonial medical establishment did not win popular support for its vaccination efforts in Burma.

## *The Vaccination Department*

The major obstacles to expanding vaccination operations were administrative disorganisation and poor funding.[1] This was perhaps unavoidable given the lack of uniformity in Burma's colonial administrative structure, a result of the gradual organisation and reorganisation of the colony after the three Anglo-Burmese wars. Until 1862, when the Province of British Burma was officially created, what was known as Lower Burma consisted of three separate colonies, each under a different administration. Even after the annexation of Upper Burma in 1886, the British exercised only limited control in large areas nominally under them, such as the Shan states.

Despite decades of British rule and efforts at vaccination since the 1830s, a sustained government initiative to introduce the procedure began only in 1864. In 1863, when Captain H. Nelson Davies wrote to the Chief Commissioner of British Burma, Colonel H. M. Durand, on the extension of vaccination in Pegu, he observed that despite frequent attempts, the results "have only been partial" and were confined to a limited number of large stations which had civil surgeons or indigenous medical staff.[2]

A contributing factor was that Burma was not the most attractive station for colonial medical officers and it was difficult to get sufficient European (or Indian) doctors or apothecaries to staff the stations in the province. Medical officers sent to Lower Burma came from the IMS and included British physicians and Indians who had received adequate medical training in their country. Burma was not a desirable posting among members of the service and the Government of India frequently complained it was difficult to find medical officers who were willing to serve in the colony,

1 Bhattacharya, Harrison, and Worboys examine administrative devolution in relation to the complexities in the discourse on the vaccination establishment on the subcontinent. Bhattacharya, Harrison, and Worboys, *Fractured States*.

2 1/1 (A) Accession 609, 1863, File no. 45, "Extension of Vaccination in British Burma", Box 1863 (2), Letter from Captain H. Nelson Davies, Secretary to the Chief Commissioner, British Burma, and Agent to the Governor General, to Colonel H.M. Durand CB, Secretary to the Governor of India, Foreign Department, Governor General's Headquarters at Calcutta, dated Rangoon, 2 May 1863, NAUM, 4.

where living conditions for those in government service were poorer than in India. This problem worsened during the 1860s when "native" (Indian) doctors from medical institutions in India chose not to go into government service.[3]

Efforts were made to extend vaccination operations throughout the province, including its remote interior. Edward Green Balfour (1813–1889), a surgeon and the acting Deputy Inspector-General of Hospitals in British Burma, proposed appointing a circuit superintendent and two assistants in Rangoon and Maulmain, where they would be in charge of the circuits of both the towns and their immediate hinterland. This proposal was approved and implemented by the colonial government in 1864. Nevertheless, these were only two towns and medical officers had to be seconded from British military regiments stationed near other Burmese towns to serve as civil surgeons. Vaccination work in the other towns thus became one of the many responsibilities (military and civil) assigned to beleaguered civil surgeons. They repeatedly suggested that a vaccination department be founded to provide proper European supervision through superintendents who would devote their time exclusively to the extension of vaccination. Sub-assistant Surgeon Bhuttacherjee, the Superintendent of Vaccination in Rangoon, urged the government to establish a well-organised vaccination agency similar to the one in British India. The civil surgeon in Thayetmyo, J. M. Miller, charged the government with poor support for vaccination. He wrote in his report on Thayetmyo in 1867–68 that he had requested vaccinators several times but the authorities had paid no heed. So, the substantial burden of vaccination and other work at the dispensary had to be borne entirely by him and one native doctor.[4]

[3] 1/1 (A) Accession 859, 1867, File no. 70, Box 1867 (3), W. A. Green, Memorandum, to the Secretary to the Government of India, in the Home Department, no. 1748B, dated 5 February 1867, NAUM, 5.

[4] 1/1 (A) Accession 609, 1863, File no. 45, "Extension of Vaccination in British Burma", Box 1863 (2), Letter from Captain H. Nelson Davies, Secretary to the Chief Commissioner, British Burma, and Agent to the Governor General, to Colonel H. M. Durand CB, Secretary to the Governor of India, Foreign Department, Governor General's Headquarters at Calcutta, dated Rangoon, 2 May 1863, NAUM, 4, 5; *Report on Vaccination for 1868*, appendix, xxii; *RVB for 1867–68*, 13, 39.

Funding had a decisive impact on the evolution of vaccination operations in Burma. It determined the scope of the operations, the number and quality of personnel used for them and, indirectly, their overall success. The colonial desire to gain the most at the least cost to imperial funds delayed government efforts to vaccinate a significant portion of Burma's population. In 1866, Chief Commissioner Phayre lamented that he could allow only one health officer each to officiate in Maulmain, Rangoon, and Akyab due to "the uncertainty as to funds" and no one in other towns though he realised a health officer was necessary in each one of them. Further, he depended on municipal funds to provide for the health officers in Maulmain and Rangoon, while in Akyab, half the cost had to come from the "bazaar" fund. As for other towns, he had to find sufficient local funds to pay for the health officers if they were to be appointed.[5] The civil surgeon in Toungoo, Charles Parker, attempted to draw the attention of the government to the funding situation the following year.

> The question of expense is of course one which it is not my province to touch upon, but I think money spent in introducing vaccination into British Burma, in a systematic and general manner, would be well laid out, and the obstacles not greater if so great as those which have been successfully overcome in the Presidency of Madras.[6]

The main reason the Government of India was so unenthusiastic about establishing a better-organised vaccination agency was the budget. The district vaccinators' costs were defrayed from the imperial revenue. The 1868 vaccination report for Maulmain reveals how costly vaccination operations in Burma were.

> [To] vaccinators who receive a fixed stipend . . . may be attributed the . . . result that an establishment of one Superintendent and four Vaccinators costing the State annually Rupees 1,800 was unable to vaccinate more people than 535. Every successful case in Maulmain has cost the Province no less than Rupees 3-14-7.[7]

5 1/1 (A) Accession 778, 1866, File no. 237, "Public Health", 1866 (4), Minute by the Chief Commissioner, British Burma, Camp at Pounglay, district of Prome, dated 27 February 1866, 10–11.

6 *RVB for 1867–68*, 42.

7 *Report on Vaccination for 1868*, 23.

Finally, in the same year, vaccination operations in Burma were brought under a special department with the establishment of the Vaccination Department. The government sanctioned the appointment of a superintendent of vaccination in Burma in September 1868. At the same time, district vaccinators were appointed, funded from the imperial revenue, and they were to be under the direct supervision of the superintendent. Along with this, the large towns of the province received varying numbers of vaccinators, who were to be under the tutelage of the local civil surgeon and funded by each municipality.

TABLE 3: Vaccination Staff During the First Decade of Operations, 1867–77

| *Year* | *Special "Native" Superintendents of Vaccination* | *Vaccinators* | | | *Total "Native" Establishment* |
|---|---|---|---|---|---|
| | | *1st class* | *2nd class* | *Total* | |
| 1867–68 | 3 | no bifurcation | | 20 | 23 |
| 1868 only | 2 | | | 20 | 22 |
| 1869–70 | 2 | 8 | 10 | 18 | 20 |
| 1870–71 | 2 | 8 | 22 | 30 | 32 |
| 1871–72 | 2 | n.a. | n.a. | 24 | 26 |
| 1872–73 | 2 | n.a. | n.a. | 24 | 26 |
| 1873–74 | 2 | n.a. | n.a. | 24 | 26 |
| 1874–75 | 2 | n.a. | n.a. | 29 | 31 |
| 1875–76 | 2 | 10 | 20 | 30 | 32 |
| 1876–77 | 2 | 10 | 21 | 31 | 33 |

*Source*: Administration and vaccination reports for the years listed.

The newly organised Vaccination Department, however, did not solve all the problems associated with the administration of vaccination operations despite the hopes of the Government of India. The 1868 reforms that created the department did give civil surgeons control over vaccinators employed in their stations but they were not given any powers to test "the correctness" of indigenous vaccinators' returns.[8] As mentioned, civil surgeons already had

[8] *RVB for 1869–70*, 154.

time-consuming responsibilities such as running the dispensary and their stations. They now had to be in charge of vaccinators and their work as well. This was a difficult, even impossible, task because they had to be at the dispensary and could not personally accompany vaccinators into the field to check on their work and progress. So the vaccination returns submitted to them by indigenous vaccinators were treated with a high degree of scepticism by the British medical authorities. In Bassein, civil surgeon Nisbet could not check the vaccination returns made by a Burmese candidate for the post of vaccinator in 1868 because his operations had been conducted "too far from the station". Village officials who might have authenticated this candidate's report showed no inclination to cooperate. In addition, the civil surgeons had to serve as medical officers to the regiments near their stations and the military work often claimed much of their time. At Thayetmyo, for example, Miller excused his unsatisfactory vaccination returns by pointing to the extra military medical work he did.[9]

The ineffectiveness of the new Vaccination Department was also partly due to inadequate funds and medical supplies, at least outside Rangoon. The consequences of this were seen during a smallpox outbreak in Prome in 1869. The town's Burmese residents asked civil surgeon Cowie to build "a special Small Pox Hospital", which would isolate all the smallpox patients from the healthy population. Cowie was dismissive of the possibility of doing so, saying "we have not the means at hand in the shape of establishment, to conduct such an Institution". He also lamented that the medical establishment in Prome was in a dismal state, with even the dispensary not having the necessary medicines. Abandoned by the Vaccination Department, the people of Prome took preventive measures into their own hands. They built barriers of wood across the streets in villages where smallpox patients were concentrated so that the healthy would be aware of the danger.[10]

Funding was a perpetual headache for the British medical authorities. The funds allocated to each district were never enough to pay for the ambitious task of extending vaccination from scratch. The limitations imposed by a meagre budget even prompted civil

9 *RABB during 1867–68*, 167; *RVB for 1867–68*, 23.

10 *RPHVS for 1869*, appendix, vii.

surgeon Donnelly to call for more generous spending on the grounds that it would be a good investment for the future.

> But vaccination is still in its infancy; and that state of every enterprise is costly. By and by the average cost of each successful case ought not to be more than a couple of annas. As the work expands, however, I cannot doubt but that the sum required from the public purse will be far in excess of that now allotted for the purpose. An anticipation which is far from being a gloomy one; for in these days every one is prepared to admit that in no other investment of its capital can a country expect such a profitable return as from that expended upon well-considered schemes for the improvement of the public health.[11]

At the same time, there was much resentment and frustration over the role of indigenous vaccinators, who, many colonial medical officers felt, were not cost effective. Donnelly was appalled by the unsatisfactory results produced by the indigenous vaccinators in Maulmain. They were vaccinating Burmese at an average cost of over three rupees per person. He reproached the vaccinators, pointing out they "receive a fixed stipend instead of having to earn their bread by the sweat of their faces". Referring to the outrageously high rate paid for each successful vaccination in Maulmain, he sarcastically remarked, "At such a rate the wealthiest and most enlightened country in the world would shrink from the duty of vaccinating its people".[12]

The Vaccination Department's expenses were normally met from provincial funds and local and municipal corporation funds. In 1876, about half its budget was contributed by the provincial fund and the rest by local governments and municipalities. Though the municipal contribution was initially considered to be very little, local funding increased by the end of the nineteenth century and contributed about half the cost of all operations. This may have exhausted local funds because it was reported that the provincial fund was increasing its share to cover a decrease in local funding from 1897. After the annexation of Upper Burma in 1886, imperial funds were allotted to meet the increased cost of vaccination operations, which had grown beyond the scope of district funds.[13]

11 *Report on Vaccination for 1868*, 13.

12 Ibid., 23.

13 *RABB during 1876–77*, 161; *RABB during 1877–78*, 76; *RABB during 1897–98*, 96; *RABB during 1895–96*, 90.

The formation of the Vaccination Department created as many problems as it solved. Its early failures were due to two main factors. First, funding remained minimal and civil surgeons found vaccination efforts hampered by a continuing shortage of money. Rather than negotiating with one source of funding, they had to wrestle with three different sources, all of which attempted to minimise their contributions. This problem was gradually solved over the course of the next few decades as the colony and local municipalities became wealthier, and smallpox deaths mounted. Second, the vaccination operations performed by "native" vaccinators remained unsatisfactory. It was not until the early twentieth century that such operations improved substantially. More about that follows.

## *Early Indigenisation of the Vaccination Staff*

As early as 1863, civil surgeons found that "native" vaccinators could supplement their vaccination work by taking over a good deal of the legwork involved.[14] They also expected that "native" vaccinators would aid operations in Burma in another important way—by acting as mediators between them and the indigenous population. "Native" vaccinators, it was hoped, would move around from village to village in the interior that overburdened civil surgeons could not visit, convincing the population about the benefits of vaccination. They would thus expand the horizon of colonial control to remote areas. However, these plans failed in many cases. The most important obstacle was at the very source of these efforts. Burmese vaccinators suffered from a lack of training and education, leading colonial medical authorities to characterise them as ignorant and neglectful. As a result, rather than trusted "native" intermediaries between the civil surgeons and the indigenous population, what emerged was a class of "native" vaccinators disrespected by both the colonial medical authorities and the Burmese people.

[14] *RABB during 1862–63*, 4; It was reported that in 1867, when the overcrowded portions of the town of Rangoon were hit by smallpox, "several native doctors and inoculators, have applied to the civil surgeon for lymph and instructions, and have commenced to aid him as vaccinators". *RABB during 1866–67*, 82.

Almost as soon as "native" vaccinators were employed, however, colonial medical authorities began what proved to be a long series of attempts to blame them for failed vaccination operations. The ethnicity of vaccinators was the first major issue. There was a growing belief, justified in some ways, that the Burmese were reluctant to accept non-Burmese vaccinators because of cultural differences and the inability of Indian vaccinators to communicate with them in Burmese. In 1868, for example, a civil surgeon concluded that the returns of vaccinators who were Indians were "not creditable" and that "their place must now be filled by Natives of the district". In Prome, a "foreign" vaccinator named Tunao, whose ethnicity remains unknown, was reported to have caused many failures in vaccination. He was replaced in 1869 by "a respectable Burman", who was later said to have greatly improved the situation. In Henzada, the number of vaccinations almost doubled from 480 in 1866–67 to 797 in 1867–68. A report gave credit for this to a "native" doctor who worked as a vaccinator. In Tavoy as well, when the colonial medical authorities appointed a Burmese named Shway Oh as a vaccinator, there was an improvement in the returns. C. W. Street, the Deputy Commissioner of Prome, requested the Commissioner of Pegu to send a Burmese vaccinator from Rangoon, saying, "The Vaccinator should if possible be a Burman—he would have greater influence, perhaps one could be sent up from Rangoon". In Prome, in 1868, when two Burmese vaccinators, Maung Shway Tha and another Burman, resigned, leaving only an Indian in place, the number of vaccinations dropped. Or so the civil surgeons would have us believe. In an attempt to find an easy excuse for the slow pace of vaccination, the failures of Indian vaccinators were emphasised while those of Burmese vaccinators, though noted and sometimes mildly criticised, did not enter the general discourse as a significant problem. For instance, the report for 1867 said that a Burman assistant vaccinator, Maung Pho, could only persuade 215 people to get vaccinated in Rangoon, far lower than the previous year's 800. This drop was merely mentioned, without any explanation, presumably assuming that Maung Pho's ethnicity was sufficient reason for the lower number, ignoring the possibility that he could have been very incompetent.[15]

15 *Report on Vaccination for 1868*, xxi, 14; *RVB for 1867–68*, 16, 33.

Determining who was and who was not "Burmese" also presented some complications. Religion was not considered a priority, for Muslim vaccinators were hired on the basis that they had Burmese mothers. When the Vaccination Department wanted to replace an Indian vaccinator who was reportedly disliked by the Burmese, the move was opposed by the *ex officio* superintendents on the basis that his mother was a native of Arakan and he "was consequently as nearly a native of the country as the Arakanese themselves". Confident that Burmese or Indo-Burmese vaccinators, not Indian ones, would solve their problems, the civil surgeons encouraged a complete shift to indigenous Burmese vaccinators. In the vaccination report for 1869–70, the names of Burmese vaccinators can be seen in almost every medical station in British Burma, ranked as first-class or second-class vaccinators under civil surgeons. There was now an indigenous vaccinator assigned to each village circle (a basic unit of rural administration in colonial Burma).[16]

Once "native" was redefined as solely Burmese and not broadly Indian and Burmese, the problems that emerged could not be excused on the basis of ethnicity alone. As discussed earlier, the quality of lymph played a significant part in determining the outcome of operations. But the Western medical faith in vaccination was such that colonial medical officers ignored questions concerning the quality of lymph while reporting the progress of the vaccination programme. They were more likely to blame indigenous vaccinators for incompetence than the lymph when operations failed. There were a number of cases in which indigenous vaccinators were accused of handling the vaccine incorrectly, and it was sometimes reported that they mixed the vaccine lymph with smallpox virus. On other occasions, some vaccinators were accused of not being careful in guarding the vaccine paste from direct exposure to the sun, whose heat nullified the lymph's efficacy altogether.[17] Burmese

16 In Pegu division, Moung Shoey Bay and Tsan Dine, Poh Kyeen in Rangoon, Pho Moung and Poh Kin in Prome, Nga Hpo Thing in Myanoung, Moung Khine in Bassein and Moung Pain in Toungoo. In Tenasserim division, Kyah Ming, Showy Mow, Bah Sin and Shway Bwa in Maulmain, Moung Shoey Moe in Shwegyeen, Shoey Oh in Tavoy and Shoey Htoon in Mergui. In Arakan division, Tha Doke Kyne in Akyab and Shoey Phai in Sandoway. *RVB for 1869–70*, 4–5. These vaccinators received a salary of either £3 or £2 a month. *RABB during 1869–70*, 154.

17 *RPHVS for 1869*, 48; *NSVB for 1903–04*, 3.

vaccinator Meer Mahomed, for example, was blamed for the failure of the lymph in his possession. "Lymph that was found good in other stations proved worthless in the hands of Meer Mahomed".[18] In 1868, just a year after a number of Burmese volunteered to aid vaccination operations, the British medical officer stated,

> As soon as the Native Vaccinator attached to the dispensaries goes out into the district away from the civil surgeon, his returns become untrustworthy, and no reliance can be placed in his work, as often or not he inoculates the children brought to him with some vile disease.[19]

In Prome, civil surgeon MacDonald blamed the poor rate of success in his district on both the ignorance of vaccinators and the lack of good lymph, "owing to the same ignorance which rendered the vaccinators unable to make a judicious selection of subjects from whom to obtain it".[20] In the vaccination report for 1871–72, it is clear that the colonial medical authorities distrusted Burmese vaccinators. Superintendent of Vaccination Kelly remarked, "Generally speaking all Burman Vaccinators required constant supervision and urging to get them to exert themselves, and it has become apparent that it is utterly vain to expect them to do any work when away from it".[21] Nearly 30 years later, these views continued to hold sway. Little, the Superintendent General of Vaccination in Burma, complained in 1902 about a "lazy vaccinator" who would revaccinate his adult friends or enter their names as revaccinated to make up for his negligence in vaccinating children in the area under his charge, submitting figures that his superior officers had no way of verifying.[22]

Medical officers also began to make personal attacks on native vaccinators on grounds of alleged immorality. In an explanation for the falling off of vaccination numbers in the Arakan hill tracts, for example, a medical officer blamed the native vaccinator for negligence. He added that this vaccinator "was lately found to be habitually gambling with bad characters",[23] as if the British could demand that all native vaccinators behave morally. Worse still

18 *RVB for 1869–70*, 5.
19 *RABB during 1868–69*, 130.
20 *Report on Vaccination for 1868*, 17.
21 *RVB for 1871–72*, 9.
22 *TRVB for 1899–1900–1901–02*, 3.
23 *NSVB for 1896–97*, 1.

was insubordination. There were some occasions when native vaccinators were said to have deliberately neglected their work. In Mandalay, the civil surgeon speculated that disgruntled indigenous vaccinators, who resented the appointment of an assistant superintendent of vaccination, caused a large drop in vaccination numbers in 1893, though no evidence of intentional insubordination was provided.[24]

While British medical authorities made long lists of the faults of their indigenous vaccinators, they inadvertently revealed their own faults as well. Bhuttacherjee, the Superintendent of Vaccination in Rangoon, wrote that the indigenous vaccinators "were taught the various modes of operations". But the amount of teaching done was debatable. The little information available on vaccinator training indicates there was no thorough or systematic approach. According to Bhuttacherjee himself, his indigenous vaccinators served as dressers in the dispensary and learned "some of the practical branches of the Medical Science" during the rainy season, a time they could not conduct vaccinations.[25] Whatever the training involved, and whether British or Indian doctors were able to surmount the language barrier, it does not seem to have gone far enough. At the very least, there was a lack of responsible training for indigenous vaccinators. For example, Kelly pointed out that indigenous vaccinators were ignorant of how to vaccinate and how to distinguish between good and bad vaccine. One civil surgeon pointed to the way they incorrectly referred to all vaccinations followed by unsuccessful vaccinations as revaccinations.[26] The cases of mixing vaccine lymph with smallpox virus or carelessly exposing the vaccine paste to direct sunlight also seem to suggest that indigenous vaccinators were not adequately trained. Little explained,

> The experienced or well-instructed vaccinator should be able to discriminate with accuracy the perfect vesicle and the typical cicatrix of successful vaccination, from spurious or unsuccessful results. The lesson is not very difficult to learn . . .[27]

The obvious question is if the lesson was not difficult to learn, then why were the indigenous vaccinators unaware of it? The

24 *RABB during 1893–94*, 93.
25 *RVB for 1867–68*, 17.
26 *RVB for 1870–71*, 9; *RABB during 1895–96*, 89.
27 *TRVB for 1899–1900–1901–02*, 2.

medical authorities continued to blame the vaccinators rather than their lack of training.

The colonial doctors considered one reason for the failure to be "the class of persons who can be had as Vaccinators".[28] Burmese vaccinators were mostly uneducated, inexperienced, and under-trained, and the villagers who knew the backgrounds of these vaccinators had little confidence in them. The civil surgeon in Prome reported that some Burmese villagers "have openly remarked that they did not consider the Vaccinator more skilful than an ordinary coolie".[29] Civil surgeons believed that a contributing factor was the high turnover among the ranks of the vaccination staff. After they partially stopped employing indigenous doctors and inoculators as vaccinators, they relied on any Burmese who volunteered. However, the Burmese, according to the Prome civil surgeon, were an "indifferent class of men who seek employment, as vaccinators", and they were quick to resign if "pressed in the matter of work". In sum, as Little pointed out, the condition of the vaccination establishment in Burma was that it was "badly educated, badly paid, and badly disciplined".[30]

## *Supervision*

From roughly 1870, the civil surgeons' discourse on the failures of the vaccination campaign focused on improving the operations and returns of the indigenous vaccinators. The Government of India and the chief commissioner were well aware of the necessity for regular inspection and verification. They requested all civil officers, to engage in

> personally ascertaining the truth or otherwise of the recorded results, and testing on every possible occasion the soundness and purity of operations performed, and in no case should a Vaccinator be allowed to proceed into the interior of the District until the Superintendent has satisfied himself that he is thoroughly competent for the work which he has to perform.[31]

28 *RVB for 1867–68*, 36.
29 *Report on Vaccination for 1868*, appendix, xxi, xxx.
30 *NSVB for 1902–03*, 1; *NSVB for 1903–04*, 1.
31 *Report on Vaccination for 1868*, iii.

A civil surgeon's report said how many vaccinations had been conducted, how many of them had been successful, and compared these numbers with those of the previous year. It also speculated on the reasons for the increase or decrease in numbers, and had some remarks on the operation, including an evaluation of the vaccinators and the reactions of the indigenous population. A civil surgeon could only contribute what he saw from the vantage point of the urban station he was in. For information on operations in rural areas (and even within the town if his duties there were onerous), he had to depend on the returns submitted by the indigenous vaccinators. Civil surgeons had a certain degree of trust in the accuracy of reports made about vaccination operations close to their stations. But they and other medical authorities lost faith in the returns when vaccinators went "on tour" to the interior.[32]

This lack of faith prevailed on all rungs of the administrative ladder. Civil officers who summarised civil surgeons' reports in their district or provincial reports meant for the Government of India had to resort to guesswork to assess the state of vaccination in areas under their jurisdiction. Most of their observations were constructed from pieces of information gathered by vaccinators who, in many cases, were not trusted. Many civil officers doubted the correctness of the data they received and suspected indifference on the part of their vaccinators. They offered suppositions and speculation that added to the confusion about what was really happening in the villages and in some towns and municipalities. Suggestions for the improvement of the accuracy of vaccination returns included changing the criteria for successful and unsuccessful vaccinations. Untrained vaccinators were classifying cases that developed sores and eruptions after vaccination as successful, even though they were not. Rather than sort out the mess this produced in the registers, in 1869, civil surgeon MacDonald suggested treating all such cases as unsuccessful.[33] Much more than such "bandage" measures, however, was needed.

The great fear of medical and civil authorities was that poor work by the indigenous vaccinators would give vaccination a bad name. Careless vaccinations would lead to more suspicion and distrust among a people who had already been encouraged by inoculators

32 *RABB during 1867–68*, 165.

33 *RPHVS for 1869*, appendix, vi.

to be wary of the operation.[34] The authorities fully believed that there had to be European supervision of the vaccination work undertaken by native vaccinators in remote areas. They had already found that superintendents were useful in managing indigenous vaccinators in the field. In 1868, two European superintendents had been appointed in Rangoon and Maulmain and, in the 1870s, the Vaccination Department began to appoint superintendents from among the Burmese. These indigenous superintendents were hired on the same principle "native" vaccinators had been hired—they were inexpensive supplementary labour and it was assumed that they would be better able to negotiate with other "native" people (in this case, "native" vaccinators).

Their introduction, like so many other reform efforts, did not solve the problem of questionable returns. There were always wide variations among the reports of different vaccinators in terms of average numbers and costs. While some indigenous vaccinators appeared to perform poorly, there were a few others who apparently did well. Whether this was due to misrepresentation in their returns or actual differences in skill and commitment was a question that remained unanswered, even with native superintendents monitoring them. The indigenous vaccinator in Kyaukpyu, for example, performed three times more successful vaccinations than his counterparts in Rangoon and Hanthawaddy in 1881.[35]

Colonial medical authorities confronted the difficulties of supervision by creating more posts for indigenous superintendents of vaccination. However, these efforts continued to focus on classroom merit, not performance in the field. In 1905, R. MaCrae, the Superintendent General of Vaccination in Burma, began a reorganisation scheme that would see more Burmese superintendents of vaccination appointed to more districts. Every three vaccinators were to have one indigenous superintendent supervising their work. In 1908, the inspector-general of civil hospitals issued an order that limited the civil surgeon's responsibility and power to verify vaccination reports, making it easier for Burmese superintendents to manipulate their returns of verification work. Entrican complained that civil surgeons were no longer allowed to inspect vaccination cases and this meant greater

34 *RABB during 1867–68*, 165.
35 *RABB during 1881–82*, 128.

TABLE 4: Vaccination Establishment, 1898–1931

| *Year* | *District Superintendents of Vaccination* | *"Native" Supervising Officers* | | | | *Vaccinators* |
|---|---|---|---|---|---|---|
| | | *Sub-Assistant Surgeons* | *Public Health Inspectors* | *Superintendents of vaccination* | *Head Vaccinators* | |
| 1898–99 | unavailable | — | — | 12 | — | 186 |
| 1899–1900 | 38 | — | — | 14 | — | 195 |
| 1900–01 | 38 | — | — | 14 | — | 192 |
| 1901–02 | 38 | — | — | 14 | — | 194 |
| 1902–03 | 38 | — | — | 15 | — | 213 |
| 1903–04 | 39 | — | — | 15 | — | 224 |
| 1904–05 | 40 | — | — | 16 | — | 233 |
| 1905–06 | unavailable | — | — | 16 | — | 241 |
| 1906–07 | unavailable | — | — | 32 | — | 211 |
| 1907–08 | unavailable | — | — | 44 | — | 253 |
| 1908–09 | 41 | — | — | 48 | — | 259 |
| 1909–10 | 41 | — | — | 48 | — | 266 |
| 1910–11 | 41 | — | — | 49 | — | 268 |
| 1911–12 | 41 | — | — | 49 | — | 269 |
| 1912–13 | 41 | — | — | 49 | — | 272 |
| 1913–14 | 41 | — | — | 44 | — | 278 |
| 1914–15 | 41 | 5 | — | 44 | — | 280 |
| 1915–16 | 41 | 22 | — | 41 | — | 297 |
| 1916–17 | 42 | 24 | — | 38 | 3 | 299 |
| 1917–18 | 42 | 26 | — | 38 | 3 | 308 |
| 1918–19 | 42 | 28 | — | 39 | 3 | 321 |
| 1919–20 | 43 | 29 | — | 41 | 3 | 325 |
| 1920–21 | 41 | 29 | — | 46 | 3 | 347 |
| 1921–22 | 41 | 35 | — | 46 | 3 | 337 |
| 1922–23 | 41 | 31 | — | 43 | 1 | 336 |
| 1923–24 | 41 | 36 | — | 44 | 1 | 337 |
| 1924–25 | 41 | 27 | 6 | 43 | 1 | 342 |
| 1925–26 | 41 | 27 | 8 | 44 | 1 | 365 |
| 1926–27 | 41 | 27 | 9 | 42 | 1 | 377 |
| 1927–28 | 41 | 28 | 11 | 43 | 1 | 384 |
| 1928–29 | 41 | 31 | 13 | 42 | 3 | 385 |
| 1929–30 | 41 | 31 | 13 | 40 | 3 | 392 |
| 1930–31 | 40 | 32 | 26 | 41 | 3 | 396 |

*Source*: Administrative and vaccination reports for the years stated.

reliance on indigenous supervision.[36] To deter any deviation from departmental standards, the colonial medical authorities threatened indigenous vaccinators and superintendents with tougher measures, including imprisonment, and sometimes invoked them.

Oversights in the departmental reorganisation scheme allowed and even made possible corrupt activities. The problem was that government vaccinators were not allowed to charge a fee for their services while private vaccinators were entitled to do so. This obviously gave poorly paid government vaccinators an incentive to pretend that they were private vaccinators. Without some sort of visible identification, villagers could not tell the difference. The cost also made poverty-stricken villagers shun vaccination operations. As Entrican observed, on the basis of information from Reverend Ferguson, even villagers who were willing to undergo vaccination could not afford to do so. They therefore resorted to inoculating their children. In addition, the government's new appointment system also seems to have created a climate for indigenous vaccinators to neglect their work. Entrican pointed out that the appointment system created great resentment among indigenous vaccinators because superintendents were appointed and put up for promotion based on their performance in a written examination. Many vaccinators who energetically conducted vaccinations, but failed the paper examination, were deprived of the opportunity of becoming superintendents.[37] On the other hand, those who were able to become indigenous superintendents were automatically granted promotions and increased pay on the basis of seniority. The 1911 description said,

> The system of appointing any person a Native Superintendent who has passed the necessary examination, and of not promoting an old and trustworthy vaccinator to the post has taken from the vaccinator all hope of promotion to a higher grade. It has left the country with a class of Native Superintendents of Vaccination who are young and inexperienced and in some cases unreliable, and who rise to a higher grade not by merit but at the expiration of every five years' service.[38]

It is not too difficult to understand why indigenous vaccinators, denied the possibility of promotion, began to seek out other ways

[36] *TRVB for 1902–03 to 1904–05*, 1; *TRVB for 1908–09 to 1910–11*, 5–6, 8.
[37] *TRVB for 1908–1909 to 1910–1911*, 8.
[38] Ibid.

of making money. This involved various forms of misconduct such as falsifying travelling allowance reports and selling vaccine lymph to inoculators. In 1911, Entrican reported that attempts were being made to convince the provincial government to open up more opportunities for indigenous vaccinators who had been sidelined and to regrade superintendents of vaccination on the basis of merit as well as length of service.[39]

Blame for the failure of vaccination operations was also occasionally laid at the doors of civil surgeons. After the opening of the Meiktila training school in 1906, for example, British medical authorities began to focus on their civil surgeons' lack of enthusiasm or interest in their work. Civil surgeons had been criticised for slackness and laziness in the past. Donnelly said in 1868,

> The Civil Surgeon himself is responsible . . . Medical Officers appoint their own Vaccinators, and it is their duty to instruct them . . . I cannot see the faintest shadow of an excuse for their omitting to train them for the duties.[40]

However, poorly motivated civil surgeons could always blame their vaccinators, whose returns and operations were not seen directly by the higher level civil and medical authorities. Civil surgeons frequently excused themselves from vaccination work they were involved in because of their responsibilities in the hospitals and dispensaries. They explained that they could not leave their stations for 10 days or so at a time to inspect vaccination work in the interior because the difficult Burmese terrain ruled out making quick tours. Discourse on the failures of vaccination, which could no longer be blamed simply on the quality of the lymph or the vaccinators, now included additional issues such as the difference in the amount of verification work carried out by the civil surgeons. In 1912, for instance, while the figure for the civil surgeon in Sandoway was more than 70 per cent, it was only 48 per cent for the civil surgeon in Prome.[41] In other words, responsibility for vaccination efforts now shifted from training (or the handling of lymph) to civil surgeons, who were held accountable for failures under their watch. If the vaccinators were doing a poor job, it was because the

[39] Ibid.

[40] *Report on Vaccination for 1868*, 17.

[41] *TRVB for 1908–09 to 1910–11*, 5–6; *NSVB for 1912–13*, 2.

civil surgeon was not doing his. Improving the performance of civil surgeons was a more difficult problem than dealing with indigenous vaccinators or even lymph. Some civil surgeons were prosecuted in the 1890s on the charge of incompetence, but such cases were few.

Deputy sanitary commissioners were supposed to help out with the inspection work that the civil surgeons were unable to do. However, they were few in number and were in charge of "the whole of Burma which covers an area of 236,738 square miles",[42] which made it an impractical arrangement. This left the responsibility for the inspection of vaccination solely in the hands of the indigenous superintendents, who British medical men such as Entrican believed to be mostly incapable men. By 1911, there were calls that the Government of India approve hiring more deputy sanitary commissioners for Burma. The shortfall in numbers was made worse by a decline in the availability of British medical staff during and after World War I. District medical officers frequently had to leave for military service in Europe or the Middle East. Sometimes, there was nobody available to replace those called away on military duty. In 1917, it was reported that the Vaccination Department in Burma had lost three deputy sanitary commissioners, 15 military assistant surgeons, and 13 military and civil sub-assistant surgeons to the war effort.[43]

As a result of the increasing number of trained Burmese being turned out by the Meiktila training school and the problems in obtaining medical staff from India, the colonial medical authorities in Burma adopted a localisation policy in matters to do with vaccination. In 1923, in Lower Burma, and in 1924, in Upper Burma, the district councils took over the responsibilities of supervising the vaccination staff and finding the funds to appoint them. In districts that had no councils, the Public Health Department remained in charge of the vaccinators, with funds coming from the deputy commissioner's local fund.[44]

42 *TRVB for 1908–09 to 1910–11*, 8.

43 *TRVB for 1908–09 to 1910–11*, 8; *TRVB for 1914–15 to 1916–17*, 1; *TRVB for 1917–18 to 1919–20*, 6; *NSVB for 1915–16*, 2.

44 *RAB for 1924–25*, 79–80.

## *Systematic Training*

Having generally failed in bringing about reliable supervision, the colonial medical authorities began to attempt to remove another variable by introducing more formal and systematic training for the vaccination staff. As early as 1886, the British government had sent several Burmese students to study medicine in India, hoping they would return and take charge of the outstation dispensaries, which would include vaccination work as well. To improve the quality of the vaccinators hired, the director of public instruction suggested recruiting students who had passed the seventh standard (vernacular), along with better pay and the promise of a stipend during the training period. It was even proposed that only those who could produce a certificate saying they had passed the "VI or VII standard in Vernacular education" should be appointed.[45]

By 1900, the colonial medical authorities realised that they had to have better vaccination staff quickly. But it was not until 1906, when a reorganisation of the Vaccination Department was initiated, that a substantial effort to produce truly capable vaccinators and superintendents began with the opening of a vaccination training school at the Meiktila vaccine depot. Entrican headed this training institution where indigenous candidates who wanted to work as vaccinators and superintendents of vaccination underwent "a complete course of training in theoretical and practical vaccination and in allied subjects".[46] Further, all the course work was conducted in English. King welcomed this openly, expressing his high expectations in a report,

> Seeing that this new staff will possess a fair education in English, there is a reason to hope that they will acquire such knowledge of the duties they are intended to fulfil as to prevent the occurrence of errors, which must at times be expected with the existing class of men.[47]

The course included six months of intensive training and the candidates had to pass an examination at the end of it. Only those who passed were appointed and sent out to the districts. During

45 *Report on the Administration of Lower Burma during 1885–86 and on the Administration of Upper Burma during 1886,* 63; *NSVB for 1903–04*, 3; *TRVB for 1902–03 to 1904–05*, 1.

46 *NSVB for 1905–06*, 1.

47 *NSVB for 1905–06*, 1.

the first three years, 26 superintendents of vaccination and 12 vaccinators completed the training and passed the final exam. Every year, however, there were several candidates who did not finish the course and left the school. In the initial three years, seven students dropped out, and the trend was no different in the following years. Since the government was desperate to produce better indigenous vaccination staff, the school began to provide an additional two to three months of retraining to those who did not pass the exam. Retrained candidates had to pass another exam at the end of their course.[48] From 1906 to 1923, the Meiktila school trained more than 100 native superintendents of vaccination and about 600 vaccinators. However, no matter how much the indigenous vaccination staff increased and improved, the British medical authorities decided that this training school by itself was not a solution.

From 1911, there were many cases involving the dismissal of indigenous vaccination staff. Seventeen vaccinators were dismissed in 1910–11, another 17 in 1911–12, and 13 in 1912–13. The vaccinators were accused of various wrongdoings, including falsifying returns, fraud, accepting illegal gratification, corruption, abetting inoculation (also called "connivance of inoculation"), disobedience, and neglecting their duties. Since the establishment of the training school in Meiktila, there seems to have been an increase in the number of cases of "native vaccinators" involved in anti-vaccination activities, especially cooperating with inoculators. Some vaccinators sold vaccine lymph to inoculators, who, in turn, "extort[ed] money by representing themselves as government vaccinators". A "Burman", presumably a government vaccinator, excused the residents of Shway-ok-gyaung village from vaccination in return for money and "decamped leaving behind as a register of his work, a headman's vaccination register completed 10 years earlier from Thabyechaung", a different village. By 1920, it had become apparent that the Meiktila training school had not contributed in a big way to extending vaccination in Burma. Indigenous vaccinators and superintendents of vaccination, who were graduates of the training school, were not considered especially trustworthy. Even Entrican, who headed the school,

[48] *TRVB for 1905–06 to 1907–08*, 7.

TABLE 5: Vaccination Instruction at the Meiktila Vaccine Depot and Training School, from 1 May 1906 to 1923

| *Year* | *"Native" Superintendents of Vaccination* | | *"Native" Apprentice Vaccinators* | | *District Vaccinators Under Training* |
|---|---|---|---|---|---|
| | *Under Training* | *Qualified at end of Course* | *Under Training* | *Qualified at end of Course* | |
| 1906–07 | 26 | 20 | 0 | 0 | — |
| 1907–08 | 5 | n.a. | 13 | n.a. | — |
| 1908–09 | 14 | 8 | 10 | n.a. | — |
| 1909–10 | 2 | | n.a. | 38 | — |
| 1910–11 | 3 | 2 | 39 | 34 | 116 |
| 1911–12 | 2 | — | 34 | — | — |
| 1912–13 | 4 | 4 | 32 | 31 | — |
| 1913–14 | 0 | — | 36 | 35 | — |
| 1914–15 | 5 | — | 35 | 31 | — |
| 1915–16 | 16 | 8 | 40 | 40 | — |
| 1916–17 | 2 | 2 | 41 | 41 | — |
| 1917–18 | 3 | 0 | 35 | 35 | — |
| 1918–19 | 5 | 6 | 80 | 76 | — |
| 1919–20 | | | | | — |
| 1920–21 | 13 | 9 | 44 | 43 | — |
| 1921–22 | 5 | n.a. | 71 | n.a. | — |
| 1922–23 | 0 | n.a. | 78 | n.a. | — |

reported, "The conduct of the Department can hardly be described as good". In 1921, Williams went so far as to conclude that the Meiktila school was a "failure".[49]

The training school continued for a little more than a decade after the Vaccination Department lost faith in it, the last course being provided in 1932–33.

[49] *TRVB for 1908–09 to 1910–11*, 8; *TRVB for 1917–18 to 1919–20*, 6; *NSVB for 1911–12*, 1; *NSVB for 1912–13*, 1; *NSVB for 1918–19*, 1; *NSVB for 1920–21*, 3.

TABLE 6: Vaccination Instruction at the Meiktila Vaccine Depot and Training School, from May 1923 to 1933

| *Year* | *Public Health Inspectors* | *Sanitary Inspectors* | *Sub-Assistant Surgeons* | *Apprentice Vaccinators* |
|---|---|---|---|---|
| 1923–24 | 22 | 0 | 0 | 44 |
| 1924–25 | 23 | 4 | 0 | 34 |
| 1925–26 | 13 | 0 | 0 | 56 |
| 1926–27 | 22 | 0 | 1 | 29 |
| 1927–28 | 18 | 0 | 2 | 47 |
| 1928–29 | 22 | 0 | 6 | 77 |
| 1929–30 | 0 | 0 | 0 | 87 |
| 1930–31 | 0 | 0 | 0 | 85 |
| 1931–32 | 23 | 0 | 0 | 38 |
| 1932–33 | 19 | 0 | 0 | 0 |

## *Renewed Efforts to Mobilise Indigenous Doctors*

In the late 1920s, roughly 30 years after the colonial medical establishment in Burma had rejected cooperation with native doctors in their vaccination efforts, it reinitiated attempts to learn about indigenous medicine. This does not mean that the British surrendered to indigenous medicine, for their faith remained firm in "scientific medicine".[50] However, they now realised the necessity of knowing about indigenous medicine, the medicine of the "Other", before they incorporated it into their own "scientific" practices.

There was a need for a large number of new doctors in the early 1920s due to several constitutional changes and practical problems. Burma was preparing to become a governor's province, which occurred in 1923, and, in 1922, the Public Health Board, under the Ministry of Education, which was headed by a Burmese, was created to take over responsibility of public health. Civil surgeons would no longer be in charge of public health, including all matters related to vaccination. In their place, local district councils would select and hire their own district health officers, though until they found qualified doctors, civil surgeons would be posted as the

[50] "The Burma Government Resolution on Indigenous Medicine", *Indian Medical Gazette* 63 (April, 1928), 205.

new district health officers.[51] There was also a change at this time in the government's approach to public health. Indigenous doctors were to be hired to provide free medical care to the people in local areas. As a result of these developments, the colony required a dramatic increase in new medical personnel. A small number of men for such posts came from the pool of retired civil surgeons, but there remained a large gap between demand and supply. Another development was the failure of the training school in Meiktila in the early 1920s.

To solve the problem of finding a large number of doctors at a cost that would not be prohibitive, the colonial administration turned to Entrican, the former director of the Meiktila vaccine depot. Entrican, who appears to have gained a reputation as a problem solver by successfully overcoming some of the technical difficulties associated with preserving vaccine lymph and heading the training school for vaccinators, was of the opinion that the medical establishment might be able to tap the indigenous *hseì-hsayas* (medical doctors) as a resource if they were offered a course in Western medicine. He explained,

> Keeping in mind the central and guiding principle of my proposal, that it is desirable to develop the Burman Saya, and not try and convert him into a scarecrow imitation of a European doctor, it follows the curriculum must be quite different from anything to be found in our recognised medical schools.[52]

Entrican further recommended that instruction should focus on anatomy since an understanding of the "structure and functions of the human body" was absent in the corpus of Burmese indigenous medicine. He also suggested establishing a Western medical school in Mandalay, the pre-colonial capital, where there were still a few Burmese who had formerly served as court physicians and were well versed in indigenous medicine. In 1922, the "Conference of Commissioners of Divisions and Heads of Departments" accepted

51 "Responsibilities of District Councils in Respect to Public Health Administration in Rural Areas", dated 18 September 1924, in *The Burma Hand-book of Rural Self Government* (Rangoon: Superintendent: Government Printing and Stationery, Union of Burma, 1957), 1: 138–139.

52 *Report of the Committee of Enquiry into the Indigenous System of Medicine [hereafter RCEISM]* (Rangoon: Superintendent, Government Printing and Stationary, Burma, 1951), 46.

Entrican's proposal.[53] They not only agreed to open the school in Mandalay, but also suggested opening another one in Bassein and providing stipends to the students. The pupils would be adult practitioners of indigenous medicine. For the school in Bassein, the students selected included indigenous *hsayas* such as Po Thaung, Saing, Sein Maung, Thet Shwe, Ba Shin Maung, and Hla Maung.[54] It was later reported that both these medical schools had "some success, and [that] the *sesayas* themselves [had] been keen to learn".[55]

About the same time, colonial doctors were making other efforts to introduce the Burmese to Western medicine in the vernacular. American Baptist missionaries had already done so in the mid-nineteenth century and, in the following decades, some Burmese faithfully copied extracts from Mason's translation of the *Materia Medica* into their own works. However, for decades such efforts were not sustained and a wide range of Western medical texts remained outside the reach of Burmese doctors, most of whom did not know English. The 1910s and 1920s witnessed a series of renewed attempts. At the 1910 annual meeting of the Burma branch of the British Medical Association, Burmese "Western medicine" doctors suggested that the colonial medical establishment begin translating "sanitary works and books on hygiene into Burmese".[56] However, few colonial doctors took up the task until Castor's *Nomenclature of Diseases* in Burmese in 1922.[57] This general attempt to promote Western medicine extended to vaccination propaganda

53 1/15 (C), Accession 290, 1924, File 3M-13, "Proposal for Opening Training *Sesayas* in Western Medicine at Bassein", 18, Box 10, Letter From Colonel P. Dee, MB, IMS, Inspector General of Civil Hospitals, Burma, to Commissioner, Irawaddy Division, Bassein, dated Rangoon, 16 June 1924, NAUM, 1.

54 1/15 (C), Accession number 290, 1924, File 3M-13, "Proposal for Opening Training *Sesayas* in Western Medicine at Bassein", 18, Box 10, Major W. L. Brooks, IMD, Civil Surgeon, Myaungmya, "List of Burmese *Saysayas* who are willing to undergo training in Western Medicine at Bassein", attached to letter to the Deputy Commissioner, Myaungmya, dated 2 September 1924, NAUM, 7.

55 *RCEISM*, 1.

56 "Burma Branch", *Supplement to the British Medical Journal* (30 April 1910), 194.

57 R. H. Castor, *Nomenclature of Diseases in Burmese*, Rangoon: Superintendent, Government Printing, Burma, 1922.

in the 1920s. Vernacular newspapers such as *The Burma Progress* began to publish illustrated advertisements for vaccination and postage stamps depicting vaccination as a preventive measure began to circulate in the 1930s.

In 1928, the Ministry of Education in Burma appointed a 10-member "Committee of Enquiry into the Indigenous System of Medicine". All the members were Burmese doctors and six of them had been trained in indigenous medicine. Among the four who had studied Western medicine was the chairman, Lieutenant-Colonel Ba Ket. He was a champion of Western medicine, who was known to lack confidence in the Burmese ability to absorb Western medical knowledge. He had, with a hint of cynicism, told the elite of the colonial medical establishment at the medical association meeting in 1910,

> It would be a great work to educate Burmans as has been suggested. What had taken England so many years to learn would not be learnt easily by the Burman. Teach a *loogyi* [an elder] what a germ is, and you have done a great work.[58]

Despite Ba Ket's disdain for native knowledge, the 1928 Committee received more than 500 written responses from practitioners of indigenous medicine and spoke to 61 others. The goals of the survey and interviews were

> (a) to examine and report on Burmese system of medicine (b) to consider whether Burmese system of medicine can be improved and if so in what way (c) to consider whether the training of *sesayas* should be undertaken by Government or left to private agency (d) if training by Government agency is recommended to consider:- (1) whether training should be given in Government hospitals or in a separate institution; (2) whether training should be confined to young men fresh from school, or to practising *sesayas* or should be given to both; (3) what teaching staff would be required; (4) detailed proposals regarding the length and nature of the courses, number of students and the conditions to be laid down as to educational qualifications, stipends, etc.; (5) how text books in Burmese could be provided for the use of students; (6) whether licence should be granted to successful students; (7) whether Government should prohibit unlicensed practice, and if so, after what period; (e) to consider what provision should be made for the research into Burmese medicine.[59]

58 "Burma Branch", 194.

59 *RCEISM*, 2.

On 7 June 1929, during the course of the interviews and the mailing of surveys, the government also asked the committee to find out if the Burmese population would like to have government-subsidised indigenous doctors, in the same way as retired civil surgeons and private medical practitioners were employed in places very far away from the colonial hospitals.[60]

This was an unprecedented event in colonial Burma because this was the first time that the medical establishment took indigenous medicine seriously and, more importantly, cooperated with indigenous doctors as participants in a medical discourse. Nevertheless, the substance of the enquiry was less than what it should have been and ultimately proved to be of no help to the Vaccination Department. Vaccination received little attention because the lack of government funding continued. Though the colonial medical establishment began engaging in a dialogue with indigenous medical practitioners about the transmission of Western medical knowledge to Burma, this dialogue would not include a re-evaluation of the inoculation versus vaccination debate. Despite the gradual extension of the Vaccination Acts to districts and towns and some signs that vaccination was catching on, there was neither renewed interest in the programme nor more funds to train indigenous medical doctors. In any case, the Vaccination Department unofficially made use of indigenous medical practitioners for vaccination in collaboration with missionaries, disguising these subalterns with ambiguous terms such as "private vaccinator", "medical practitioner", "private practitioner", "private medical practitioner", "private agencies", and "other agencies", all terms that did not spell out clearly that the cooperation of the Burmese was involved.[61]

## *Conclusion*

We have examined the ways in which the colonial medical establishment failed to establish a cooperative relationship with

60 Ibid.

61 *RAB for 1914–15*, 96; *RAB for 1916–17*, 109; *RAB for 1917–18*, 127; *RAB for 1919–20*, 165; *RAB for 1920–21*, 170; *RAB for 1921–22*, 148; *RAB for 1922–23*, 102; *RAB for 1923–24*, 166; *RAB for 1924–25*, 80; *RAB for 1925–26*, 87; *RAB for 1926–27*, 89; *RAB for 1927–28*, 95; *RAB for 1928–29*, 95; *RAB for 1929–30*, 100; *RAB for 1930–31*, 84, 138; *RAB for 1932–33*, 95; *RAB for 1933–34*, 116; *RAB for 1935–36*, 122.

the indigenous population of Burma, a process that required taking several complex factors into account. The authorities could not establish an effective Vaccination Department or foster the indigenous collaboration they had hoped would drastically change the medical environment of Burma. The Vaccination Department was beset with the problem of poor funding right from the start and it remained so as the Government of India shifted its financial responsibilities to various bodies at the provincial, municipal, and local levels. In addition to the department's disorganisation, the British continued to face difficulties in obtaining accurate information from the indigenous vaccinators, and in winning the confidence of the Burmese people. Their attempts to overcome these difficulties by indigenising the vaccination staff and educating them at the newly opened training school in Meiktila only created further problems. A new appointment system for native superintendents of vaccination scotched all hopes many indigenous vaccinators had of being promoted, tempting them to supplement their income through illegal activities and collaboration with inoculators. Native superintendents of vaccination were also corrupt, the powers of civil surgeons over them being curtailed. Thus the colonial medical establishment in Burma could not produce indigenous agents to help promote vaccination. This lost the Vaccination Department its best chance to extend vaccination in the province. In 1928, the British assembled a committee to inquire into the indigenous system of medicine in the hope that they could mobilise Burmese medical doctors, the very people whom they had ignored, ridiculed, and disregarded for almost a century.

By relying increasingly on an indigenous vaccination staff, which the colonial medical authorities found hard to trust, an elaborate administrative machine was set up, which repeatedly failed but continued to grow. As a result, though vaccination operations expanded in the early twentieth century to a level unimagined a few years before, the sheer scale of the new operations ensured that problems and obstacles also dramatically increased. At a time when Britain was facing popular resistance from the Burmese in other ways, the vaccination establishment frequently lost confidence in the eventual success of its programme.

# 7

# *Vaccination Legislation*

The editors of the *Maulmain Chronicle* complained in January 1842 that the local vaccination campaign against smallpox was in danger of coming to a close. It was suggested that the number of people willing to be vaccinated was declining, presumably because faith in the procedure had not spread beyond the Europeans. The editors suggested that the authorities be pressured to force vaccination among the indigenous population by making it compulsory for Burmese children.[1] This became a reality in colonial Burma roughly 40 years later. The development of medical policy on smallpox and other contagious diseases in Burma was informed by the health policies in Britain, something the colonial government found was very effective for consolidating its power over the general population. While the public in Britain resisted the state's expanding control over health and the body by claiming to be "conscientious objectors", the colonial government allowed no such escape for the people of Burma. As other measures failed to achieve complete victory over smallpox, the colonial medical authorities increasingly relied on legislation to help them in their fight. Furnivall once identified the colonial state in Burma with "leviathan".[2] Reflecting his model of ever increasing state power, the health authorities in Burma steadily attempted, quite often successfully, to enhance their legal powers and authority over the Burmese to push the vaccination agenda forward. We will examine the discourse on increasing legal authority among colonial medical officers, the tensions that emerged between municipal civil authorities and health authorities over the growing power of health officers, and

[1] *Maulmain Chronicle* (26 January 1842).

[2] J. S. Furnivall, *The Fashioning of Leviathon: The Beginnings of British Rule in Burma*, edited by Gehan Wijeyewardene (Canberra: Australian National University, 1991).

the immigration of Indian coolies who were identified as the source of smallpox outbreaks. All these elements contributed to the growth of state power through health legislation.

## *The Pursuit of Legal Authority*

As early as 1867, there were active exchanges of opinion over the issue of prohibiting inoculation and making vaccination compulsory in Burma. Supporters and opponents argued, citing legislative obligations and responsibility, Burma's social conditions, the dangers of inoculation, the progress of vaccination, and numerous other related matters. Frustrated with the glacial progress of vaccination, some civil medical officers and government authorities accused the legislature of neglecting the interests of the population and urged it to enact the necessary legislation without hesitation. In 1868, Benjamin Thomas Suffrein, who had been the civil surgeon in Toungoo (1863) and Prome (1864–1866) and at the time was officiating as the civil surgeon in Maulmain, emerged as a strong advocate of legally enforced vaccination. He recommended that parents be required to obtain a certificate of vaccination for children under the age of one. Such a law was necessary to extend vaccination in Burma, he argued, because the indigenous population was not yet "enlightened". Even in "enlightened" England, he observed, there were some parents, belonging to the "intelligent" middle or upper classes, who were averse to submitting to the law and refused to have their children vaccinated. On the other hand, in "unenlightened" Burma, which he implied consisted only of the lower classes, one could see even uneducated parents opposing vaccination. So, he argued, the government needed to prohibit inoculation and force those Burmese to undergo vaccination by law.[3] Likewise, Nisbet's 1869 treatise on vaccination and inoculation pointed out how effective a law on vaccination had been in contemporary Prussia.

> Take the history of the operation in Prussia, and throughout Germany, North and South. There the operation is enforced by law, and has been for nearly half a century. And what has been the result? It may be told in three words. Small-pox is extinct. In the Small-pox Hospitals in various parts of Europe, where the disease is not yet stamped out in this energetic way, the preventive power of vaccination is displayed in a very

[3] *Report on Vaccination for 1868*, appendix, xxx.

marked way. In those ghastly abodes of suffering humanity, vaccination of the hospital attendants is as strictly carried out, as it is in Prussia, from a different cause, viz, from their natural fear of contagion. The result is that not a single death from Small-pox has been recorded for the last 20 years amongst those thus habitually exposed to the contagion.[4]

An 1870 report summed up the view of G. E. Marr, the civil surgeon in Maulmain, another strong advocate of enforcing compulsory vaccination in Burma. He observed that nothing like "perfect success" had attended vaccination in "countries where the legislature has not stepped into assistance by rendering its acceptance compulsory and the practice of inoculation penal".[5]

Many colonial medical authorities, however, opposed legislation enforcing vaccination. Cowie, the civil surgeon in charge of the Rangoon Charitable Dispensary, spoke out in 1867 against any law prohibiting inoculation because he believed that vaccination was yet to find its feet in Burma. In 1868, Lieutenant Colonel E. M. Ryan, while officiating as the Commissioner of Tenasserim, raised a different point of view regarding the relevance of such laws to Burma. He argued that it was true the province was in an "uncivilised" stage of national development and, for this reason, the laws would not work.[6] Other colonial doctors disagreed with legislative solutions on the grounds that vaccination was not yet a perfect solution. Donnelly, the Superintendent of Vaccination in British Burma, also came out against the prohibition of inoculation in 1868. The poor performance of the colonial vaccination programme, he argued, made it unwise to ban inoculation. It would be cruel to force the Burmese to abandon inoculation, their only "safeguard" against smallpox, and would be the same as telling them to perish. Moreover, any move made against inoculation, he predicted, would raise resistance to future efforts to spread vaccination.

> In a low state of civilisation national customs present to the people very much the same aspect as their religious institutions, and any attempt to interfere with them is regarded as the act of an enemy and in the light of persecution.[7]

[4] Ibid., appendix, xvii.
[5] *RVB for 1869–70*, 30–31.
[6] *RPHVS for 1867*, 37–38; *Report on Vaccination for 1868*, appendix, xxvi.
[7] *Report on Vaccination for 1868*, 25.

This could result in the colonial cause of vaccination in Burma running into quicksand, he warned, "rendering all the British propaganda about the benefit of vaccination suspicious for Burman eyes".[8]

At the end of the 1860s, doctors who favoured delaying the ban on inoculation shared the opinion that the colonial government's reach outside Rangoon was too weak to make vaccination a wholly reliable alternative to inoculation. Donnelly argued that bringing effective vaccination to Burma was beyond the financial capacity of the government.[9] Laws by themselves would also do little, he pointed out. Using the example of Nisbet's 1869 argument that vaccination had succeeded in Prussia because of the "vigorous interference of the State", Donnelly contended that this kind of government intervention, which was backed by Prussia's "despotic government that interferes with every act of a citizen", was not possible in most of British Burma. The medical establishment in Burma was also not in a state to provide full attention to vaccination throughout the entire colony. Cowie, the first Sanitary Commissioner for British Burma, added,

> The difficulty in this country . . . is to "bring effective vaccination" to the doors of the people, and secondly the "effective supervision" so necessary in this practice is totally wanting.[10]

The obvious compromise was to apply such a law only to places where colonial control was firmly established and pervasive, he said, which meant that it could only be enforced in those villages and towns where vaccination had already been successfully propagated among the indigenous population.[11]

## *The British Model*

The idea of using legislation in the fight against smallpox in Burma was informed by the legislative experience in Britain. There, under the Vaccination Acts issued in 1853, 1867, and 1871, the so-called Poor Law Guardians had to take steps to vaccinate all infants in districts under their charge—independently until 1858 and with

8 Ibid., 25.

9 Ibid., 24

10 *RPHVS for 1869*, 47–48.

11 Ibid., 47–48.

the Medical Department of the Privy Council after that. Though these laws operated on the pretext of providing free vaccination to the poor, in reality, they forced parents to get their children vaccinated. Porter and Porter discuss the ways in which the Medical Department of the Privy Council expanded its power while enforcing compulsory vaccination. Medical officers such as John Simon believed the problem of extending vaccination had much to do with "the system of medical management", where the Poor Law Board's powers to supervise its implementation were limited. Simon initiated changes which became the foundation of the new Vaccination Act of 1867. This Act made it compulsory for children under the age of 14 to be vaccinated and parents who neglected to do this faced fines or imprisonment. It also encouraged doctors and newly appointed Vaccination Officers to enforce the law and notify the defaulters. These provisions "further extended to an unprecedented degree state powers of compulsion".[12] Coercive vaccination measures became "a political innovation" to consolidate state authority over the "body" of the general population.

Enforcement of smallpox vaccination was resented in nineteenth and early twentieth-century England (as it would be in Burma), and in the metropole, led to violent opposition in the form of a popular anti-vaccination movement. Nadja Durbach argues that this movement was mobilised not only by its middle-class leadership, which saw the Act as a transgression on individual liberty, but also "by members of a large and politically active working class who argued against state interference with their own bodies".[13] Many workers were pressured by their employers to have their babies vaccinated, for an unvaccinated baby could spread smallpox among workers from otherwise healthy families. The working-class anti-vaccination activists separated themselves from "a lower stratum of uninformed, negligent, or lazy parents", whom they labelled "undeserving" paupers, and distinguished themselves as "'respectable' and 'conscientious' citizens".[14] This "citizenship",

[12] Porter and Porter, "The Politics of Prevention", 232–33.

[13] Nadja Durbach, "'They Might As Well Brand Us': Working-Class Resistance to Vaccination in Victorian England", *Social History of Medicine* 13, no. 1 (April 2000), 46.

[14] Ibid.

Durbach explains, was regarded as a privilege derived from English citizenship and was not regarded as a universal human right.

Nineteenth-century Britain created a rich collection of legislative models for fighting smallpox in British India. The colonial medical authorities drew on some of them, such as the laws requiring compulsory vaccination. But the circumstances in Burma made it inevitable there were differences in the way they were implemented. In the face of growing opposition to the 1867 Act among large segments of the metropolitan population, the British government caved in, recognising the parental right to refuse adherence to the Act on the grounds of conscientious objection. While the people of "a lower stratum" in Britain were able to use the logic of conscientious citizenship to oppose vaccination, the Burmese could do no such thing. They simply remained indifferent to vaccination while undergoing inoculation. The colonial government in Burma did not respond positively to indigenous passive opposition. Nor was opposition in the metropole taken into account. Rather, it intensified coercive measures to spread vaccination in Burma.

## *Legislation in Burma*

While the anti-vaccination movement was gathering force in metropolitan Britain, the colonial authorities enforced a similar Vaccination Act in Burma in 1880. In British India, as Arnold points out, there were some sections pressing the government to make vaccination compulsory. They were the advocates of modernising India, who claimed that the colonial government was obliged to protect the health of its subjects through vaccination. The Government of India, however, was not enthusiastic about taking hasty measures to enforce vaccination because it was not sure what the reaction of the "unenlightened masses" would be.[15] Though colonial health policies elsewhere in British India were replicated in Burma, there were some differences in the ways in which vaccination was enforced. Religion, the caste system, and the length and degree of colonisation were all factors that contributed to this.

15 Arnold, *Colonizing the Body*, 154.

The first major step towards legislative support for vaccination in Burma was the Vaccination Act of 1880. The Act gave municipalities and cantonments the "power to prohibit inoculation and to make the vaccination of children compulsory".[16] But the Act's introduction to districts and towns occurred very slowly. Initially, the municipal committees in Rangoon, Toungoo, and Akyab applied to extend the Act to their towns, though Toungoo quickly withdrew its application.[17] The Akyab municipal committee met with strong opposition from the people and postponed its proposal until suitable arrangements could be made. In Rangoon, vaccination services were not efficiently organised and there was no consensus on introducing the Act because the honorary magistrate and the municipal committee had not yet discussed the issue. In Prome, local opinion was sharply divided and there was strong opposition to the extension of the Act. The Prome municipal committee's decision to apply the law took a decade, until 1890, and the vote was extremely close, those in favour numbering seven to five.[18] The slow pace at which the Act of 1880 gained municipal approval (see figures 9.1, 9.2, and 9.3) can be discerned from the fact that it took three years for it to be promulgated for the first time in Burma, by the Akyab municipality. Rangoon followed suit in 1884, Maulmain in 1885, Bassein in 1888, Henzada, Hawkareik, Myanaung, Thayetmyo, and Toungoo in 1889, and Ngathainggyaung-Daunggyi, Paungde, Prome and Sandoway in 1890. All these towns were in Lower Burma. The Act was not extended to any town, municipality, or cantonment in Upper Burma until March 1891, mainly because of ongoing resistance to the British annexation of 1 January 1886. Even decades later, it had not been fully extended to some Burmese towns.[19] District councils did not extend the Vaccination Act to rural areas under their jurisdiction until 1924.[20]

16 Act No. XIII of 1880 (9 July 1880), in *The Burma Hand-book of Rural Self Government* (Rangoon: Superintendent, Government Printing and Stationery, Union of Burma, 1957), 1: 135.

17 The report does not explain why this decision was made. *RABB during 1881–82*, 127.

18 *RABB during 1881–82*, 127–128; "Vaccination in British Burma", *British Medical Journal* 1 (27 May 1882), 791.

19 *RABB during 1890–91*, 93.

20 *NSVB for 1924–25*, 3–4.

Many colonial doctors in Burma believed that the vaccination law helped the cause of vaccination in Burma, albeit without much Burmese enthusiasm. In 1893, it was reported that vaccination was making good progress, with 110,149 vaccinations performed in Upper Burma and 156,116 in Lower Burma. By 1898, Surgeon-Colonel Sinclair felt comfortable lauding the rapid advance of vaccination in the province.[21] Regardless of actual improvement in vaccination operations, these numbers only appeared in British administrative reports, British medical journals, and English newspapers. They were meant to be seen, judged, and appreciated only by the colonial government and not meant to be seen and understood by the general population. For indigenous Burmese outside the small, English-speaking elite, these numbers meant very little, for few would have been aware that statistics of any kind were being kept.

## *Municipal and Popular Resistance*

Since the 1880s, the increasing powers of the colonial medical authorities gave rise to resentment, which eventually flared into open resistance, among both local civil authorities and the general population. With their legislative powers and constitutional control of local government, municipal authorities presented a serious legal obstacle to the medical establishment, especially when it came to compulsory vaccination. Though the civil authorities feared smallpox and went along with the civil surgeons in supporting the Vaccination Act of 1880, they also harboured fears about the safety of the operation. Moreover, they were interested in limiting the effect of any measure that would hamper commercial activities. So they were reluctant to concede any powers to the provincial medical authorities beyond those already granted by the 1880 Act. This was illustrated by the Rangoon municipality's decision on the "German Club incident". On 21 August 1896, a complaint sent by the secretary of the German Club to H. L. Eales, the municipal president (1896, 1897–99), was read before a public meeting of the council. The secretary urged a municipal investigation into an incident that had taken place and included the account of an eyewitness.

21 "Vaccination in Burma", *British Medical Journal* 1 (2 April 1898), 927–28.

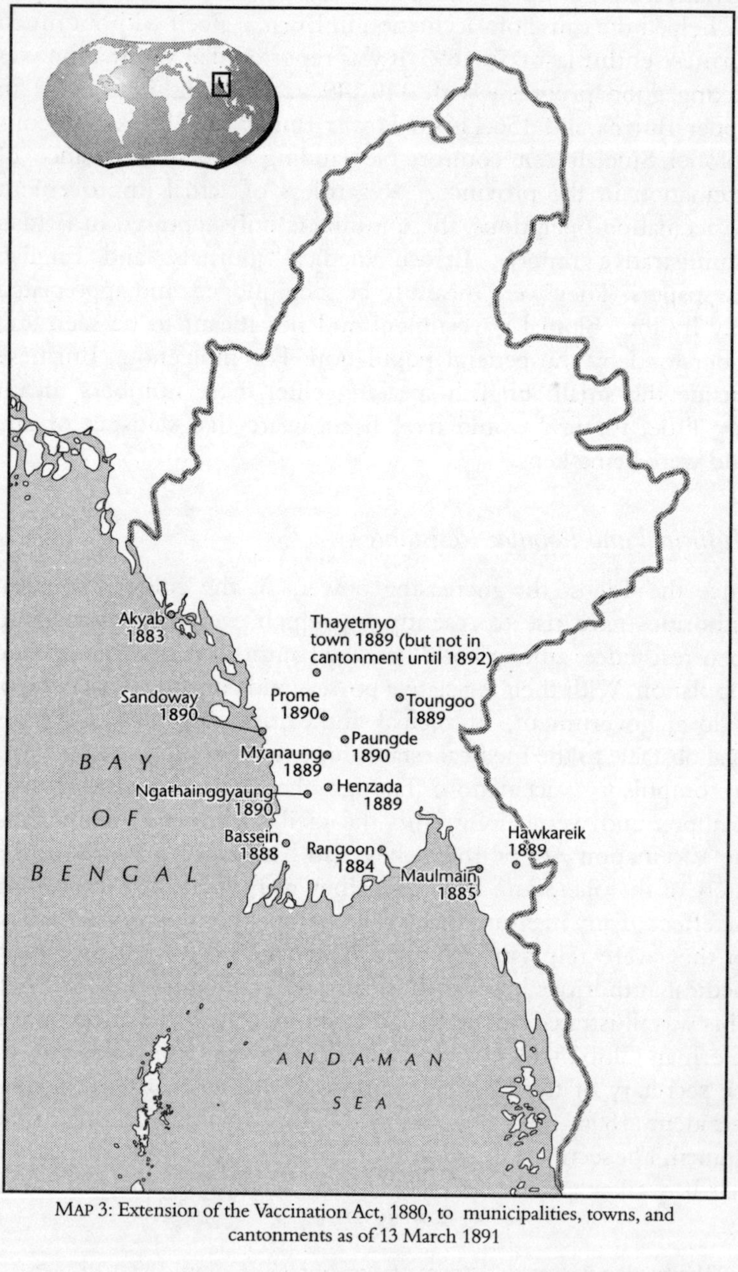


MAP 3: Extension of the Vaccination Act, 1880, to municipalities, towns, and cantonments as of 13 March 1891

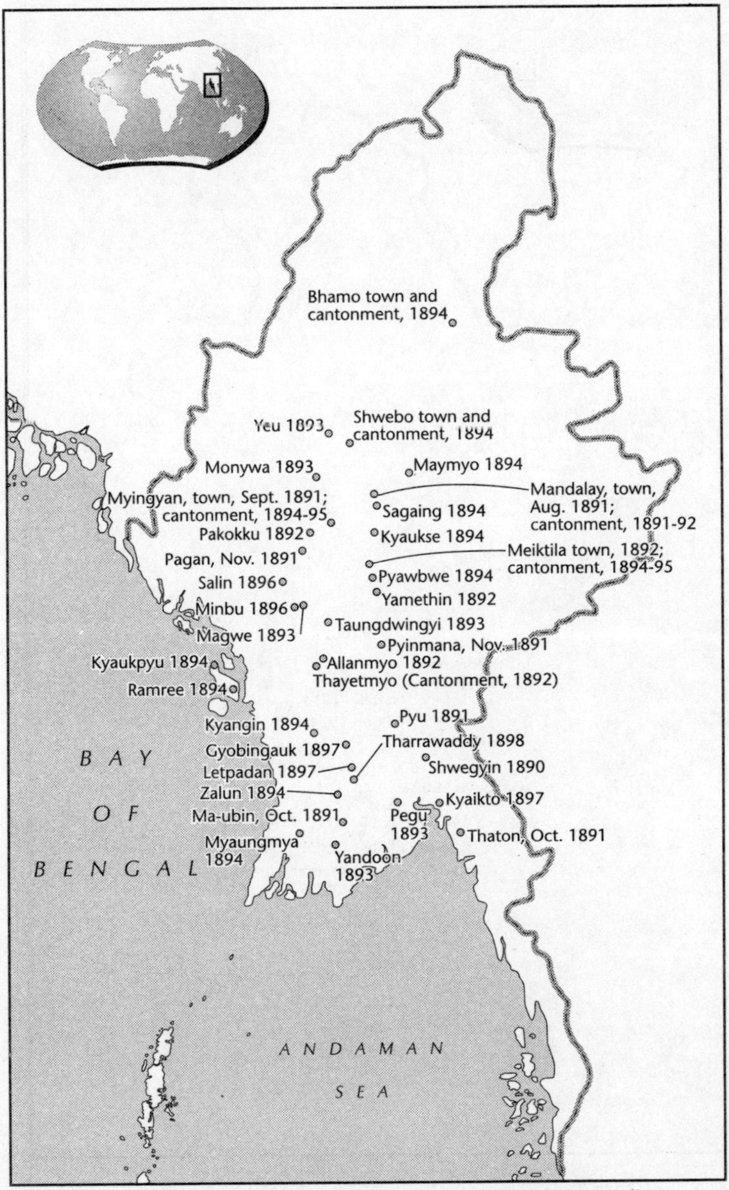


MAP 4: Extension of the Vaccination Act, 1880, to additional municipalities, towns and cantonments from 14 May 1891 to 1900

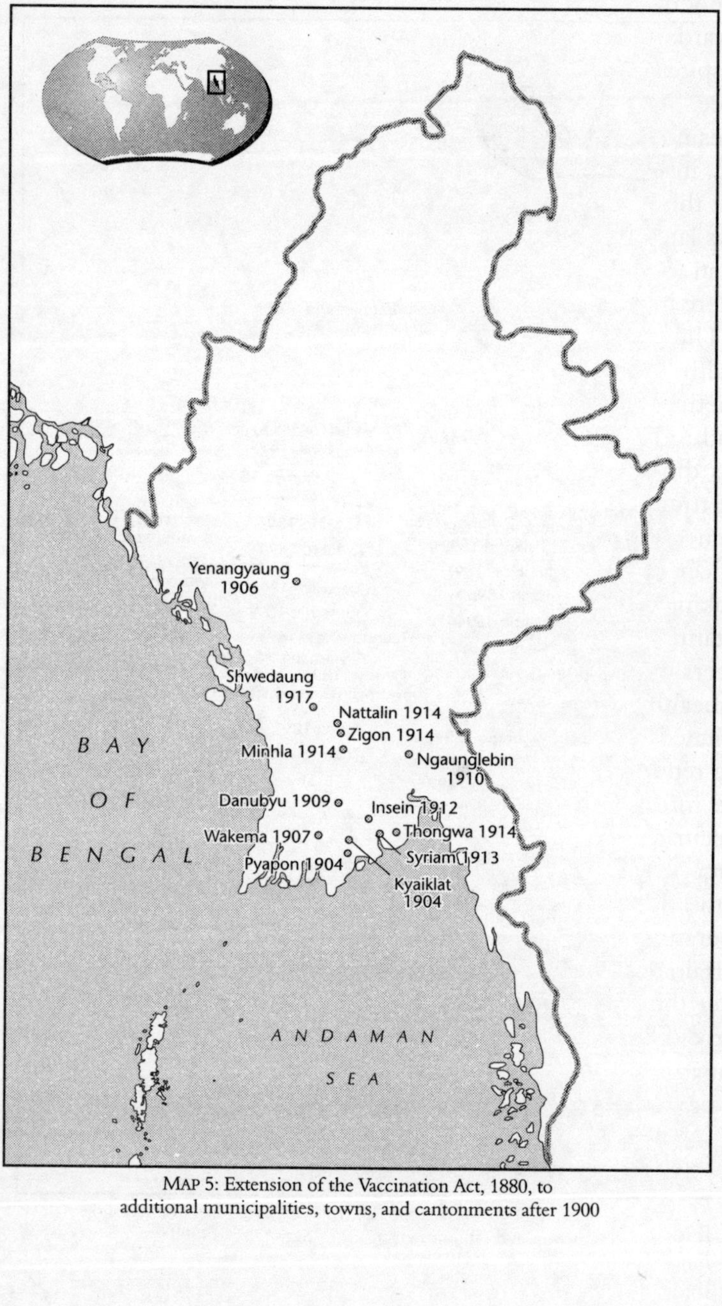


MAP 5: Extension of the Vaccination Act, 1880, to additional municipalities, towns, and cantonments after 1900

The letter said that when three servants of the club were walking towards it, they were stopped by staff at the vaccination depot. Despite their refusal to accept vaccination, they were vaccinated by force. Soon after the operation, "one of the Burmans" (the report gives no other information as to his identity) approached a servant and inspected his vaccinated arm. This Burman, "pretending" that the servant "was not properly vaccinated", did it again. Three days later, this servant developed a high fever and tetanus. He was taken to the health officer, who ordered that he be sent to hospital, where he died two days later.[22]

The secretary said in the letter that he was appalled municipal health officers had used such force. He enquired, "May I ask whether Municipal servants are allowed to force people on the road to be vaccinated against their will?"[23] By the time the matter was discussed before a meeting of the hospital subcommittee of the municipal council on 26 September 1896, an investigation had been carried out and it was reported that the municipal health officer determined the cause of death had been "two unhealthy looking ulcers on his arm in the usual vaccination position". Tetanus, it was asserted, had entered the system through these ulcers due to lack of care by the deceased, since "after vaccination unhealthy ulcers were liable to form if the site of vaccination was irritated by dirt and exposed to the air".[24] During discussions on the report, a councilman named Wagoner said that it was possible the infection had been caused by dirty instruments used by the vaccinator. His main concern, however, was "the unnecessary force used".[25] Eales informed the meeting that he was aware that some doctors recommended compulsion to conduct vaccination operations and that for some time vaccinators had been employing a certain degree of "gentle persuasion". However, due to uncertainty over the cause of infection and concern over the use of excessive force, he sided with the secretary of the German Club. The order issued was displayed on public boards and said that "nobody was to be vaccinated against his will and that no charge was to be made

22 *Rangoon Gazette and Weekly Budget* (21 August 1896), 5.

23 Ibid.

24 *Rangoon Gazette and Weekly Budget* (26 September 1896).

25 Ibid.

for vaccination so that a check would be put upon the vaccinator's zeal". In effect, it nullified the Vaccination Act of 1880.[26]

The concern revealed in letters published in the *Rangoon Gazette* was that the municipal health officers had violated personal autonomy. However, the municipal health officer evaded this critical issue in his report, probably because he resented being bypassed by the municipal council. He focused on the municipal president's order banning compulsory vaccination, which, he claimed, would make Rangoon susceptible to smallpox brought in by the Indian coolies pouring into town. The health officer argued that it was negligence on the part of the German Club servant that had caused the secondary infection, which led to his death. The officer claimed the servant had made some kind of paste with leaves and dirt containing the tetanus virus and applied it to the vaccination vesicles. Going beyond medical explanations, he diverted attention to public reaction, complaining to the authorities in Calcutta and London that Eales's orders had "produced such a scare in the popular mind".[27]

Whether the municipal president's ban on compulsory adult vaccination was politically motivated or not, it came in the way of protection from smallpox in the overcrowded port-capital. The colonial health authorities were outraged and expressed their fears about Indian immigrant "coolies", who were unscreened, and thus presumably unprotected from smallpox. The municipal health officer observed in his report that the authority of health officers in Rangoon had suffered, and "no adult coolies who keep constantly pouring into Rangoon in large numbers could be persuaded to submit to the operation".[28]

In terms of public acceptance, the success of the 1880 Act seems to have been less real than apparent. Being forced to accept vaccination did not win over the popular mind and, as one report mentioned in 1893, "the attitude of the people towards vaccination is described as generally antagonistic".[29] Burmese began leaving the municipalities where vaccination was enforced, accounting for

26 Ibid.

27 *NSVB for 1896–97*, 8; *RABB during 1897–98*, 96.

28 *NSVB for 1896–97*, 8.

29 "Vaccination in Burma", *British Medical Journal* 1 (5 March 1894), 499.

a decrease in the number of vaccinations in some towns. A civil surgeon in Lower Burma reported,

> They fully understand that vaccination is not compulsory outside municipal limits, nor inoculation illegal, so that villages which willingly submitted to vaccination in past years had been aloof altogether on one pretext or another.[30]

Thus the limited nature of the law provided the Burmese with ways to circumvent government authority. As Donnelly had speculated earlier, a simpler though more far-reaching law would be needed to undermine native faith in inoculation.

The Burmese flight from vaccination revealed the limitations of the 1880 Vaccination Act. The Act was promulgated only in municipalities, towns, and cantonments, thus excluding rural areas and, hence, the majority of the Burmese population.[31] Some areas, such as the Shan states in north-eastern Burma, were beyond the law altogether and it was reported that vaccination was making little headway there because "the mass of the people are indifferent if not hostile".[32] Colonial doctors began to argue that the 1880 Act would not work, and vaccination would fail if it was not extended to rural areas. Some unrealistically argued that doing so would make little difference to the Burmese. Entrican, for example, advocated extending the Act to rural areas, arguing that the rural population would not resist it because of their "ignorance". He explained, "I think that it would meet with no opposition, in fact the majority of villagers would never know or realise that any change had been made".[33]

While the new health measures introduced by the Epidemic Diseases Act of 1897 were so strict that they "provoked the greatest upsurge of public resistance to Western medicine and sanitation" in India, the Burmese reaction was slower and more circumspect. For some time, it was largely confined to Rangoon, the colony's most important port, though MaCrae, the Superintendent General of Vaccination in Burma, reported that the population was generally hostile to the new measures. The hostility in Rangoon, where

30 *NSVB for 1902–03*, 1.

31 R. Grant Brown, *Burma as I Saw It. 1889–1917: With a Chapter on Recent Events* (London: Methuen, 1926), 157.

32 *RABB during 1890–91*, 93.

33 *TRVB for 1917–1918 to 1919–1920*, 6.

1,706 people were prosecuted in 1905, was probably linked to the increased vaccination activity that took place during a major outbreak of smallpox in 1905–06. The disease caused 8,540 deaths in 1906 and vaccinations during 1905–06 were 45,450, almost double the figure for 1904–05 (24,081), a smallpox-free year in Rangoon.[34]

## *Class and Health Segregation*

New health legislation also coincided with emerging communal self-awareness and national identity, especially since it reflected the increasing stratification of colonial society, particularly in Rangoon. With the encouragement of the Government of India, there was a large influx of Indian immigrants, especially from Madras, into Burma. This input to sustain and support the rapidly growing rice export economy contributed to the changing ethnic makeup of Rangoon.[35] As the European and Eurasian population grew, and the rich among the Chinese, Indians, and Burmese identified themselves as members of the colonial elite, there was a growing Burmese and Indian working underclass that resented inequalities in the application of the law, including medical legislation. These disparities were revealed during the outbreaks of plague and smallpox in 1905–06, a crisis that led to a blending of the powers provided by the Epidemic Diseases Act of 1897 and the Burma Vaccination Law Amendment Act of 1900. The overlapping epidemics resulted in special camps for their victims and other strict measures, but all this did not apply equally to all classes.

Segregation camps for smallpox, plague, and cholera patients were arranged, both to accommodate the large number of cases and to move the sick far away so that they could be prevented from spreading the diseases. During the decade before the 1905 outbreaks of plague and smallpox, the Rangoon municipality had moved towards more specialised facilities for the treatment of contagious diseases. An 1896 report claimed, referring to the Rangoon General Hospital, that the "accommodation for infectious disease is unsuitable and inadequate", even though the town also had a general contagious diseases hospital and a special smallpox

[34] *TRVB for 1902–03 to 1904–05*, 5; *NSVB for 1906–07*, 2.

[35] Richell, *Disease and Demography in Colonial Burma*, 30–32.

hospital. In 1899, Rangoon municipality president H. L. Tilly urged borrowing money so that a new contagious diseases hospital could be built in the Kandawgalay ward, consisting of two sub-hospitals, one for Europeans and the other for "natives". As more and more people became infected with plague and smallpox, as well as cholera, Rangoon and other municipalities and towns found their hospitals were bursting at the seams and created isolation camps. Though a variety of names were used, these camps fell into two main categories, the contagious camps for the victims of disease and the segregation camps for those who had come into contact with victims or lived in close proximity to them, but were not infected. Maulmain erected epidemic disease sheds in Moungan, far outside town, while Tavoy set up a segregation camp in Singyubun, which was a stop for the mail steamer, thus providing convenient passage for those exposed to the plague and presumably also smallpox. In some municipalities, the large number of patients led to more specialised camps, such as the cholera camp in Thayetmyo and the separate plague and smallpox camps in Rangoon. The Rangoon smallpox camp was opened far up the Yangon river and municipal residents with symptoms of smallpox were picked off the streets by ambulances, put on board a government boat and taken to it.[36]

The conditions in these camps were appalling. In a segregation camp for smallpox in Maulmain, for example, people were accommodated in crude sheds, "which are made of bamboo and mats, structures that are not particularly comfortable". They also did not protect anyone from the "intense heat" of the midday sun, the cold wind at night, or the "damp mist" of early morning. Some of the few detailed descriptions of the poor conditions in the camps come from "accidental" cases, which involved people with close connections to the Europeans, who were able to attract the attention of English-language newspapers. One such case took place in 1906, when the treatment and death of Samuel Solomon, a Burmese Christian teacher of the English Wesleyan Mission Boys School, raised an outcry among Christian ministers in Mandalay. It all

[36] *Rangoon Gazette and Weekly Budget* (26 June 1896): 11; *Rangoon Gazette and Weekly Budget* (21 November 1896): 4; *Rangoon Gazette and Weekly Budget* (24 April 1897): 29; *Rangoon Gazette and Weekly Budget* (29 May 1899): 15–16; *Times of Burma* (9 September 1905): 5; *Times of Burma* (3 March 1906): 5–6; *Times of Burma* (17 March 1906): 12; *Times of Burma* (22 July 1905): 5.

began when a private practitioner and semi-official plague inspector in Mandalay named Kumaren investigated a reported case of the plague and found that it was actually smallpox. Since the disease was outside his authority, he informed the local health officers, who examined Solomon on the top floor of the Bible Society building and ordered that he be sent to the "contagious camp" on 73rd A Road, where smallpox victims from the town were being isolated. Solomon died of exhaustion soon after he arrived. He had been hauled in an open bullock cart under the "piercing Mandalay sun at midday", and was abandoned in an empty shed in the camp. Witnesses said that there had been no one to care for him at the camp, and no water had been available for drinking or for washing. His body was found on the ground beside a cot.[37]

Force was selectively applied to relocate people from their homes to the camps. Due to a multitude of provincial acts, amendments, municipal laws and bye-laws, measures permitted for the control of diseases (as in the case of the plague and smallpox), and a complex system of powers devolved to numerous provincial and municipal authorities, few members of the public were aware of what health officers could and could not do. At the same time that health officers in Rangoon and some other municipalities and towns were forcibly moving both plague and smallpox victims and their families to camps, residents of other municipalities and towns were calling for local and provincial legislation that would provide such powers. One, apparently European, resident of Pyinmana urged,

> The Municipality should frame some important rules in regard to the removal of a patient from any infected house to some public camp, the disinfection of houses and burning them where necessary. . . . By the Sanitary Act of 1866 in England, a penalty of £5 is inflicted on any person who wilfully or negligently is the means of spreading infectious or contagious diseases among their friends or neighbours. I don't see any reason why similar rules in Burma cannot be put in force.[38]

The permitted and appropriated powers of medical officers and the poor facilities that existed to take care of patients led to bitter complaints from the non-European communities. In Pyinmana, many plague patients and their family members refused to move

[37] *Times of Burma* (27 January 1906), 6; *Times of Burma* (3 March 1906), 5.
[38] *Times of Burma* (24 February 1906), 12.

to the segregation camp for treatment. In Rangoon, in 1906, the municipal plague staff issued an order that plague patients and their relatives in non-infected quarters be moved to a special plague segregation camp. This enraged the Muslims and "other native communities", who called a public meeting at a local mosque. The main issue seems to have been frustration with their powerlessness in the face of repeated violations of their personal space, their houses, their bodies, and their families by the government medical authorities. Special criticism was directed at the way the health officials had been disinfecting houses at will, in some cases even burning them down. Nobody wanted this to happen and, in one case, an Indian "covered with small-pox from head to foot" was taken far away and abandoned by his friends so that their barrack residence would not be fumigated. At the mosque meeting, the majority said they preferred to disinfect their houses themselves and would gladly do so if disinfecting materials were supplied to them. The meeting concluded with the threat that they would resort to force to persuade the Lieutenant-Governor to cancel the notice unless he quickly withdrew it.[39]

Generally, such non-European efforts received little sympathy in the English-language press, a factor that was responsible for delaying reform. The case of Solomon drew attention because he was a Burmese Christian, whose plight was publicised by prominent members of the local church along with threats to take the matter to the local government. One wonders how many other cases of poor treatment, involving indigenous non-Christians, went unreported in the English-language newspapers. Eventually, however, partly due to strong opposition from the people, some of the segregation camps were shut down.[40]

In contrast, the elite of the colony, Europeans and Eurasians, who lived in the cantonments, were treated better. The measures adopted in Mandalay in 1906 serve as a representative example. The medical authorities carried off the sick among the indigenous population and their immediate neighbours to the camps, but sick residents

39 *Times of Burma* (24 February 1906), 12; *Times of Burma* (3 March 1906), 6; *Times of Burma* (17 March 1906), 12.

40 *Times of Burma* (27 January 1906), 6. The segregation camp for plague patients in Sinbyubun near Tavoy was closed in 1905. *Times of Burma* (9 September 1905), 5.

of the cantonment were allowed to remain in their homes and they received individual treatment from the cantonment medical authorities. While natives who came in contact with the infected or lived close to them were sent off to segregation camps, in the cantonment, the neighbours were merely requested to decide for themselves whether they wished to relocate. Those who did, found accommodation not in the camps, but in local temples-turned-shelters within the boundaries of the cantonment. In any event, residents in the cantonments were assured they had the privilege of not being moved forcibly.[41]

## *Indian Immigrants and Vaccination Legislation*

Concerns over the perceived relationship between Indian immigration to Burma and the potential for outbreaks of epidemic diseases led to another piece of legislation, the Vaccination Law Amendment Act of 1900. The local health authorities had long identified Indian immigrants as major carriers of the smallpox virus and believed them to be the source of numerous outbreaks of the disease. Most of these immigrants were from the poorer classes and had not been vaccinated in India. Nor were they screened for smallpox when they departed Indian ports for Burma.[42] F. C. Gates, in his preface to the *Report on Vaccination in Burma for 1896–97*, reflected the general concern over the import of epidemic diseases by Indian coolies. He argued that a smallpox outbreak that had occurred in Hanthawaddy was "doubtless traceable to Rangoon Town" and the Indian immigrants there. Strict law enforcement was needed to protect the neighbouring districts, he said.[43] From the late 1890s, the colonial medical officers in Burma pursued increased authority to deal with the growing number of Indian immigrants arriving at Burmese ports, mainly

41 *Times of Burma* (17 March 1906), 12.

42 One early example offered by medical authorities was the "*Euxine* incident". In 1877, the *Euxine*, a ship carrying a large number of Indian coolies from Madras arrived at the port of Maulmain. Before departure, some of the immigrants had contracted smallpox and 20 were immediately hospitalised in the town. Only six of the immigrants died but the disease spread out of the hospital to the people of the town, causing 62 deaths within a month, and continued to spread into 1878. *RABB during 1877–78*, 74–75.

43 *NSVB for 1896–97*, 2; *RABB during 1897–98*, 96.

Rangoon, as a means of curbing the outbreak and spread of smallpox and other dangerous diseases.

Two developments encouraged an increase in the powers of the medical authorities—the smallpox epidemics in the last half of the 1890s and the outbreak of plague in India during the same period. These events brought about changes in government policy in British India generally and in Burma in particular. The attempt by Eales to ban compulsory vaccination in Rangoon, for example, indirectly aided attempts by the colonial medical authorities to gain the increased powers they sought. The consequences of the municipal ban on compulsory adult vaccination, which meant Indian immigrants avoided getting vaccinated, included a massive outbreak of smallpox in 1896 in Hanthawaddy district (referred to by Gates), followed by another in 1898–99. That the total number of deaths from smallpox in 1899 was 10,754, which was the highest figure for disease-related deaths in nineteenth-century Burma (see table 7), added particular urgency to the matter.[44]

Government concerns over the spread of smallpox by Indian immigrants also coincided with the development of health policy in British India. The widespread outbreak of plague in 1897 led the Government of India to adopt a series of emergency control measures to prevent the spread of contagious diseases. A "Plague Council" was formed in 1897 and Lord Elgin, the Governor-General of India, approved "An Act to Provide for the Better Prevention of the Spread of Dangerous Epidemic Disease", which was immediately promulgated. This gave the Indian government and the medical authorities under it extensive powers to control the plague, including the authority to check ships and passengers and destroy the houses of plague patients.[45]

British India shared a growing global concern over the movement of diseases by sea. The debate on the Bill to amend the Indian Ports Act focused on the quarantine rules for infectious diseases not

[44] Another study arrives at a different tally (7,111) for this year. See Ko Ko, Thaung and Soe Aung, "Myanmar – General Perspectives", in *Conquest of Scourges in Myanmar* (Yangon: Myanmar Academy of Medical Science, 2002), 23. It is difficult to account for this discrepancy other than suggest that these authors may be referring to only the figures for Lower Burma.

[45] Ko Ko, Thaung and Soe Aung, "Myanmar–General Perspectives", 22; Arnold, *Colonizing the Body*, 204.

TABLE 7: Deaths from Smallpox in Burma, 1891–1936

| *Year* | *Number of Deaths* | *Death Rate per 1,000* |
|---|---|---|
| 1891 | 2,363 | 0.29 |
| 1892 | 2,607 | 0.32 |
| 1893 | 5,540 | 0.68 |
| 1894 | 3,096 | 0.38 |
| 1895 | 2,770 | 0.34 |
| 1896 | 3,014 | 0.37 |
| 1897 | 3,503 | 0.43 |
| 1898 | 8,717 | 1.07 |
| 1899 | 10,754 | 1.32 |
| 1900 | 5,540 | 0.68 |
| 1901 | 3,904 | 0.46 |
| 1902 | 2,818 | 0.28 |
| 1903 | 1,952 | 0.23 |
| 1904 | 2,461 | 0.29 |
| 1905 | 1,809 | 0.10 |
| 1906 | 6,161 | 1.42 |
| 1907 | 2,882 | 0.28 |
| 1908 | 1,298 | 0.13 |
| 1909 | 1,011 | 0.15 |
| 1910 | 1,817 | 0.21 |
| 1911 | 6,004 | 0.60 |
| 1912 | 7,959 | 0.81 |
| 1913 | 2,816 | 0.29 |
| 1914 | 258 | 0.03 |
| 1915 | 217 | 0.02 |
| 1916 | 707 | 0.07 |
| 1917 | 559 | 0.06 |
| 1918 | 750 | 0.08 |
| 1919 | 3,917 | 0.40 |
| 1920 | 2,853 | 0.29 |
| 1921 | 987 | 0.09 |
| 1922 | 1,439 | 0.13 |
| 1923 | 2,846 | 0.26 |
| 1924 | 2,501 | 0.23 |
| 1925 | 3,852 | 0.36 |
| 1926 | 2,339 | 0.22 |
| 1927 | 1,704 | 0.16 |
| 1928 | 2,825 | 0.26 |
| 1929 | 1,841 | 0.17 |
| 1930 | 921 | 0.09 |
| 1931 | 490 | 0.04 |
| 1932 | 2,484 | 0.21 |
| 1933 | 1,506 | 0.124 |
| 1934 | 1,601 | 0.132 |
| 1935 | 1,262 | 0.104 |
| 1936 | 1,354 | 0.112 |

*Source*: Annual and triennial vaccination reports for the period covered.

common to India, on the one hand, and the medical inspection of those endemic to India, on the other. With regard to the second category, the Government of Madras initially made certain amendment proposals in 1888 and the Government of Bombay framed draft rules based on them, but felt that legal authority was lacking. In 1889, Lord Lansdowne, the Viceroy of India, approved the Bombay draft rules and suggested solving the problem of legal authority by issuing the rules under the authority granted by sub-section "i" of section 6, clause "p", of the Indian Ports Act. The Government of Bombay found that this legal authority did not cover all exigencies and, in 1894, brought the problem to the notice of the Indian government once again. This time, it was recommended that the Government of Bombay amend sub-section "i" so that it would cover all that was necessary for imposing the quarantine rules, or the "Medical Inspection Rules". To this end, Bombay forwarded a draft Bill in 1895, which permitted the authorities to take precautionary measures against infected vessels, including disinfecting or destroying them. The Government of India asked other "Maritime Local Governments" for their opinion and they generally agreed with the Bombay draft Bill. However, the final Bill prepared by the Government of India omitted Bombay's key provision that made it legal to destroy infected cargo, fearing it would amount to "unnecessary interference with trade". It also reduced the punishment for the infected ship's master, owner, and officers by leaving out the six months imprisonment stipulated in the Bombay draft.[46]

The port health authorities in Rangoon were unhappy that they lacked the legal authority to isolate infected vessels and their passengers.[47] Others were concerned over a clause in the Draft Rules, section 5, which said,

> When the Health Officer considers it necessary, in order to prevent the spread of disease, he may inspect the vessel, including the passengers and crew, and may arrange for the conveyance of all persons suffering or suspected by him to be suffering from such disease to a hospital,

[46] IOR/P/5798 File. No.3Z-32, from His Excellency the Governor-General of India in Council to Her Majesty's Secretary of State for India - No. 33 (Sanitary), Calcutta, 29 December 1898.

[47] IOR/P/5798, from Commander H.S. Black, Port Officer, Rangoon, to the Secretary to the Government of Burma, 7 October 1899.

unless the sick person or his friends can make adequate provision elsewhere.[48]

Understandably alarmed civil surgeons and port health officers complained that allowing a sick person or his friends to make arrangements without proper official supervision would "defeat the object of this rule".[49] Yet, it took almost a decade for an amended Indian Ports Act (1908) to emerge. The threat from an ever increasing number of immigrants pushed the authorities in port cities to seek other ways of empowering port officers to prevent the import of contagious diseases into Burma.

In its attempts to increase the powers of the health authorities as part of a comprehensive medical policy in Burma, the provincial government rapidly expanded its power over indigenous bodies. Although these particular measures were intended to control the plague, they were easily extended to the fight against smallpox and other communicable diseases. The Lepers Act, which provided for segregation in asylums, was enacted in 1898. In the same year, the provincial government proposed a new amendment to the Vaccination Act, which was enacted in 1900 as the Burma Vaccination Law Amendment Act of 1900 (Burma Act 1 of 1900).[50] The amendment clearly reflected the great concern of the medical authorities in Burma over the meagre authority granted to municipal health officers. The statement of objects and reasons for the amendment Bill stated,

> The attention of the Local Government has been drawn to the public danger arising from the dissemination of smallpox by migratory coolies, who, it is alleged, catch the disease in Burman villages and bring it to Burman towns. These coolies furnish a large percentage of the cases in Rangoon, where the disease is always more or less prevalent, and periodically approaches an epidemic stage. [51]

48 Draft Rules under section 6, sub-section (1) clause (p) sub-clause (i) of the Indian Ports Act, 1889, as amended by the Indian Ports Act 1899, for regulating the action to be taken where a vessel on which there is or has been any case of dangerous infectious disease common in India enters or is in any port subject to the Indian Ports Act 1889. IOR/P/5798.

49 IOR/P/5798, from Civil Surgeon and Port Health Officer, Maulmain, to the Deputy Commissioner, Amherst (Sanitary), 6 November 1899.

50 *NSVB for 1897–98*, ii–iii.

51 IOR/P/5798, "Bill to make further provision for compulsory Vaccination in Burma", Legislative Department-No.1150-1Z-2. From the Secretary to

Therefore, the draft Bill continued, Rangoon municipal health and port officers, as well as those of other municipalities and ports, should be granted powers to vaccinate unprotected immigrants on infected vessels, in lodging houses and in coolie barracks. The Rangoon municipal committee initially aimed to assign these responsibilities to ports of departure in the Presidency of Madras, by making vaccination compulsory for embarking immigrants. However, Madras refused to implement this scheme because of its prohibitive cost, and the Burmese authorities opposed it because of fear it would be harmful to Burma's trade and agriculture, which relied much on immigrant labour. If the Bill was passed, and its strictures imposed, it would lead to the "dissemination of absurd rumours of restrictive measures among the ignorant villagers of the various parts of the Madras Presidency from which the supply of labour mainly comes", they said. This would act as a barrier to immigration.[52] The attention immigrants from Madras were attracting had already caused the Rangoon Chamber of Commerce considerable concern. A. D. Warren, the chamber's secretary, argued that smallpox was not confined to coolies and it was "unfair to legislate for one class and not another". He further said that Indian immigrants came not only from Madras, but also other ports such as Bimlipatam, Masulipatam, Coconada, Kalingapatam, Vizgapatam and Chittagong, not to mention Singapore and Penang.[53]

The Rangoon Trade Association, on the other hand, was more vehement about controlling the import of smallpox by immigrants. Its stand was based on a report by the local health officer about recent smallpox cases in Rangoon, which stated that 2,218 cases were notified or discovered during 1898–99 and 1,413 of them had been among the natives of India. Sanitary Commissioner Sinclair was of the opinion that there was not enough proof that Indian immigrants were the main culprits. All the data available, it was suggested, could not be relied on because the Burmese, just like the Indians, were likely to conceal cases of smallpox to avoid being

---

the Government of Burma to the Secretary to the Government of India, Legislative Department, 30 March 1900.

52 Ibid.

53 IOR/P/5798, from A.D. Warren, Secretary to the Rangoon Chamber of Commerce, to the Secretary to the Government of Burma, 20 June 1899.

forcibly moved. Ultimately, the amended Vaccination Act was passed in 1900, endorsing the authority of the health officer of the municipality and port of Rangoon to vaccinate residents in coolie barracks and lodging houses.[54] However, the port authority and health officers of the Rangoon municipality were not empowered to vaccinate immigrants arriving in Rangoon on infected vessels. This was granted only with another amendment in 1909.

Indian immigrants in Rangoon soon felt the weight of the amended Vaccination Act of 1900, as well as additional legislation. The powers provided by the amended Act were put to full use during the smallpox outbreak of 1905–06. The health authorities of the Rangoon municipality carried out systematic and thorough searches of the mills, where many Indian coolies were employed, vaccinating or revaccinating 30,308 people, mostly immigrants.[55] The amendment to the amended Act gave the government more powers to suppress the contagious disease among the Indian immigrant population. In response to the second epidemic of smallpox in 1906, the government laid down the awkwardly entitled Burma Vaccination Law Amendment (Amendment) Act, 1909 (Burma Act No. 1 of 1909), also repealing the Act of 1900.[56] Though Vaccination Department authorities claimed that the 1909 amendment was merely intended to ensure that young children who were exposed to infection were vaccinated (with or without parental consent), it mandated additional measures that were easily transferable to the immigrant population. For example, it allowed health officers to order "any unprotected persons to submit to vaccination within seven days". The health authorities, including health officers, superintendents of vaccination, and other authorised officers, were given increased powers to arrest those who did not submit to this order. Even passive resistance such as not showing the physical marks (scars) of vaccination to the officers became an acceptable reason for punishment.[57]

54 IOR/P/5798, notes by Dr J. C. Hoyle, Municipal Health Officer, Rangoon, dated 9 July 1899, on the recent Smallpox Epidemic, 1898–99; IOR/P/5798, from Colonel D. Sinclair, Sanitary Commissioner, Burma, to the Secretary to the Government of Burma, 30 August 1899; *RABB during 1899–1900*, 91.

55 *NSVB for 1906–07*, 2.

56 *The Burma Hand-book of Rural Self Government*, 1:151.

57 *TRVB for 1908–09 to 1910–11*, 5.

Certain measures in the new amendment specifically addressed the issue of preventing immigrants from spreading the disease among the general population. All "labourers" who "land[ed] at Rangoon or any port to which the Local Government by notification may extend the section" were now required to proceed immediately to inspection stations where, if they were unprotected from smallpox, they would be forced to accept vaccination. Health officers conducted thorough ship searches in which they caught unreported cases of contagious diseases, including smallpox, on supposedly "healthy" vessels.[58]

As with the anti-plague and anti-smallpox efforts of the 1905–07 period and the segregation camps, the efforts to control the Indian immigrants, who were seen as primary suspects in bringing smallpox to Burma and spreading it, revealed how health legislation and policy in the colony were increasingly shaped by class. Among immigrants, the 1909 legislation targeted only deck passengers, "deck class" being the section preferred by travellers from the labouring classes. Cabin passengers, usually Europeans or wealthy Asians, were exempt. More generally, the passage of the Act meant that the medical authorities were now free to pursue members of the immigrant population wherever they worked or lived. Colonial medical officers now had permission to search and vaccinate at will, including the authority to enter private homes, "let-in" lodgings, mills, and factories.

Shortly after the 1909 amendment was enacted, colonial medical authorities attempted to focus on ships coming from Calcutta because the port was identified as a major source of smallpox. Williams, the Superintendent General of Vaccination in Burma, explained in 1917,

> The port of Rangoon is in direct steamer connection with the ports of Bengal and Madras, and hundreds of thousands of deck passengers from those Provinces, and via Calcutta, from Bihar and Orissa, the United Provinces, and the Punjab arrive annually in Rangoon. The chronological association of small-pox prevalence in Burma with epidemic outbreaks in Madras, Bengal and Bihar, and Orissa, is a close one, and during the epidemic in Madras and Bengal Presidencies many cases of the disease are landed in Rangoon, and a proportion of these come from interior parts of the two Presidencies at a time when the

[58] Ibid., 2, 5.

> ports of departure are declared free from the disease or only lightly infected.[59]

The other side of enhanced legislative powers was that they required increased medical resources. From 1880 to 1909, successive pieces of legislation widened the scope, and increased the authority, of medical officers in Burma but the situation on the ground made it impossible for them to take advantage of their new powers. Despite the reinforcement of control over immigrants, the number of Indian coolies entering Burma was overwhelming. As early as October 1909, the Burma Vaccination Law Amendment (Amendment) Act of the same year was temporarily suspended because of a shortage of accommodation at the wharf.[60] The expansion of vaccination operations and other costs also became areas of concern. The cost of taking care of the health of coolies from India fell on the shoulders of the Rangoon municipality and the Government of Burma. This included not only paying for their vaccination, but also subsidising the accommodation fees for them at the wharf, treating those who developed infectious diseases on ships, and setting up facilities for inspection. The increasing cost of health controls frustrated health officers in Burma, such as Entrican, who complained in 1921, "Practically the whole of the patients suffering from small-pox in the Contagious Disease Hospital are Indian Coolies, and the burden of looking after them falls on this Province".[61]

Though the Rangoon municipality applied the Burma Vaccination Amendment Act "somewhat spasmodically", health officers were making progress in containing smallpox at the port.[62] The number of immigrant deck passengers, all from the working class, who were vaccinated at the port of Rangoon was significant. In 1916 alone, more than 28,378 "unprotected" deck passengers, who comprised about 13 per cent of all immigrants to Burma from India that year, were vaccinated. The number of those vaccinated increased steadily: in 1917–18, 11,330 were vaccinated at the Rangoon port; 14,718 in 1920–21; 18,366 in 1921–22; 27,155

59 *TRVB for 1914–15 to 1916–17*, 2.
60 *RABB during 1909–10*, 109.
61 *TRVB for 1917–18 to 1919–20*, 3.
62 Ibid.

in 1923–24; 30,202 in 1924–25; 186,966 in 1928–29; and 216,854 in 1929–30.[63]

Despite these impressive figures, the municipal health officers still remained unconvinced of their ability to stop the spread of smallpox at Rangoon's "doorstep". Further legislation that could provide a quick solution to the evasive problem of immigrant vaccination was thus urged. Entrican, officiating as the Superintendent General of Vaccination in Burma in 1921, was convinced that vaccination measures applicable to Indian immigrants had to be further tightened. He believed that the 1909 Amendment Act did not succeed in protecting Rangoon from smallpox because it had failed to amend the definition of "protected person". The Act's definition of a "protected person" was anyone who had been successfully vaccinated at any age. This definition was outdated, Entrican argued, because a single vaccination often failed to guarantee lifetime immunity. He was concerned that many of the Indian coolies who were labelled "protected persons", according to the Act, could still be carriers of the disease and spread it to Rangoon, and thence the rest of Burma.[64] Much stricter legislation was finally enacted with the Burma Vaccination Law Amendment Act of 1928. This Act required that the Port Health Authority vaccinate all unprotected people arriving in Burma by sea unless they could prove that they posed no threat. With this Act, it was reported that "over 300,000 persons" would have to be vaccinated a year at the port of Rangoon.[65] Moreover, this Act allowed the Rangoon municipality, with the permission of the local government, to "make rules for the enforcement of the revaccination of persons having attained the age of twelve years".[66]

63 *TRVB for 1908–09 to 1910–11*, 2; *RAB for 1917–18*, 18; *RAB for 1920–21*, 171; *RAB for 1920–21*, 148; *RAB for 1923–24*, 89; *RAB for 1924–25*, 80; *RAB for 1928–29*, 95; *RAB for 1929–30*, 101.

64 As Entrican recorded, "Out of 236,139 passengers inspected only 6,455 or 2.73 per cent, were 'unprotected' in the eyes of the law, and only this handful could be vaccinated". *TRVB for 1917–18 to 1919–20*, 3.

65 Indian immigrants had to show the physical signs of having had smallpox or prove that they were successfully vaccinated or revaccinated within a period of seven years prior to their arrival in Burma. *Annual Report of the Health Officer for the City of Rangoon for the Year 1927* (Rangoon: The Burma Guardian Press, 1927), 15.

66 *The Burma Hand-book of Rural Self Government: Act and Rules* (Rangoon: Supdt., Govt. Printing and Stationary, 1957), 1: 150.

## *Conclusion*

The attempt of colonial health authorities to increase their powers through contagious disease legislation continued. In 1923, they submitted a proposal "accompanied by draft rules framed under the Epidemic Disease Act" to the government. This sought to augment the power of local authorities by adding cholera and smallpox to the plague control rules. It was a formal attempt to regularise the power health officers had periodically appropriated for themselves. In Burma, the colonial authorities attempted to take the legal route to eradicating smallpox as did their counterparts in metropole Britain. In Britain, the government faced difficulties because of public opposition to compulsory vaccination. In Burma too, the colonial government did not find it easy to follow this path, but for different reasons. The areas subject to vaccination legislation remained limited for much of the colonial period. Legislation was not extended to the rural areas until the mid-1920s. Another problem was that Indian immigrants, an ever increasing presence in the province as the rice export economy and immigration to fuel it grew, were identified as a major source of epidemic diseases, including smallpox. Richell observes that these immigrants became "whipping boys" since many of these diseases were already endemic to Burma.[67] Nevertheless, the unprecedented speed and volume of the Indian influx, and the unsanitary and crowded living conditions the coolies in big cities endured, meant that they frequently did pose a serious health threat. So the colonial government in Burma found itself facing a dilemma over changes to the Vaccination Act. It had to balance competing interests. On the one hand, it had to respond to the demands of health officers and civil officers for stricter controls to protect the health of the general population from diseases blamed on Indian immigrants. On the other hand, it had to appease the trade associations and the influential Chamber of Commerce, for whom Indian immigrants were an essential element in ensuring economic prosperity. The negotiation of these interests resulted in the Vaccination Amendment Acts of 1909 and 1928.

Legislation did provide a new means to eradicate smallpox to some degree. But making vaccination state medicine made the

[67] Richell, *Diseases and Demography in Colonial Burma*, 191.

indigenous population view it as a symbol of control to which they had to submit, a good enough reason for them to resist and avoid it. The discourse on the fight against smallpox continued to be dominated by medical officers, with no meaningful involvement of the indigenous population. Despite this, the vaccination programme in Burma finally began to move towards success in the 1920s. The standards set by the colonial-era medical authorities and the authority they appropriated for themselves were embraced by later generations of Burmese doctors. The powers granted to health authorities during the colonial period thus continued into the independence period and provided an impetus to the vaccination effort that was maintained until the end of the fight against smallpox in Burma in 1971.

# Conclusion

The first half of this study focused on vaccine lymph and the vaccine depot, examining the vicissitudes of producing and distributing effective vaccine lymph. If preventive medicine such as smallpox vaccination was intended as a "tool of empire", the lack of effective lymph rendered this tool impotent for a considerable part of the colonial period in Burma. At times, some colonial medical officers even recommended that vaccination efforts be suspended or abandoned altogether. The problem of ineffective lymph was more serious in Burma than on the subcontinent. In its early years, the Vaccination Department in Burma had to rely on bringing in lymph from the subcontinent (or Britain), and then transporting it between Rangoon and the districts in the interior. In both cases, the vaccine lymph was exposed to tropical heat, increasing the risk of it losing potency. In contrast to the subcontinent, there was no rail system in Upper Burma until the late 1880s and this made the problem worse. The second half of the study has focused on colonial attempts to win over the indigenous population to vaccination, to mobilise indigenous agents in this effort, to control indigenous inoculation, and, finally, to force indigenous "conversion" to the operation. In the process, three major sub-themes have been examined—the different kinds of knowledge that were necessary for the extension of vaccination in Burma, and the network of medical information on the cultivation of vaccine lymph; the bifurcation of the colonial landscape into urban and rural areas; and the rationality of indigenous resistance to the vaccination operation.

## *New Areas of Knowledge*

With the exception of a few studies, the role of the vaccine depot in the fight against smallpox in Burma has received little attention. Many studies look only at its formal role as a production centre for animal lymph. They generally fail to interrogate the multi-dimensional nature of its activities, for in the early stages of the evolution of this institution, its functions took it into areas of knowledge outside its stated charter. Bhattacharya, Harrison, and Worboys have looked into its forays into issues to do with the climate, the buying and selling of calves, and its research into preservatives suitable for British India. The present study adds complexity to our understanding of the colonial-era vaccine depot by looking more deeply into such issues as the considerations of topography and the more fundamental task of maintaining the animals it relied on for cultivation, testing, and experimenting. This study's examination of the Taunggyi and Meiktila vaccine depots shows unlike others, that the colonial-era vaccine depot simultaneously served as a vaccine production and distribution centre, an animal hospital, and a scientific research laboratory. It was the Meiktila vaccine depot and not other scientific research centres such as the Pasteur Institute in Burma that became the specialised institution for smallpox vaccination.

Worboys points out that there was a lack of practical incentive for bacteriological studies of smallpox in Britain after the 1880s despite the disease's importance, while there was theoretical interest in "discovering" the smallpox germ in the rich scientific milieu of germ theory.[1] At the same time, the improvement of microscopy shifted bacteriological interest in smallpox to the new research arena of culturing vaccine lymph, which followed two distinct paths. The first was towards discovering and elucidating the working of micro-organisms, and the second towards disinfecting the vaccine lymph of unwanted organisms.[2] As discussed, colonial medical officers in Burma took the initiative in this research from the late 1880s, turning the vaccine depot into an active scientific laboratory for new research into the cultivation of vaccine lymph, following a pattern also seen in the metropole. Colonial medical officers such as Entrican and King reacted to a very real need and moved

[1] Worboys has suggested that the reason for this was that "smallpox was a disease that was easily diagnosed, undeniably contagious and had a proven preventive technology". Michael Worboys, *Spreading Germs: Disease Theories and Medical Practice in Britain, 1865–1900* (Cambridge: Cambridge University Press, 2000), 244–45.

[2] Worboys, *Spreading Germs*, 244–45.

beyond the research into preservatives of vaccine lymph conducted in Europe to find the best preservative for tropical conditions, where the lymph's longevity and vulnerability to heat were major concerns. As medical officers in Burma began to look to other provinces in British India and other tropical colonies for answers, Meiktila became connected to an emerging international information network that transcended colonial boundaries. It was thus not confined to the unilateral flow of information from the imperial metropole to the colonial periphery. Research at Meiktila was increasingly conducted in communication with other vaccine institutions and depots in British India and in other European colonies such as British Malaya and the Dutch East Indies. In the process, Meiktila had its own contributions to make. It also informed the emerging international discourse on the limits of vaccine lymph vitality in the tropical context.

The shift to cow-to-arm vaccination and the cultivation of animal lymph in local vaccine depots took the medical establishment in Burma into new areas of knowledge. The vaccine depot had to procure healthy calves and maintain their health, a task that required a mild climate, a higher altitude, and access to water and grazing land. So the Vaccination Department had to carefully evaluate and assess Burma's environment as well as climatic conditions, including local temperatures, humidity, precipitation, and topography. In addition, it had to see how accessible cattle markets were for buying and selling calves, and how close the railway was to distribute the cultivated vaccine lymph quickly to other areas of the colony.

A working vaccine depot also required expertise in a new range of activities and knowledge about animals. The knowledge of cattle types increased because the vaccine depot sought "ideal cattle", defined by characteristics such as age, sex, size, and colour of hair and skin. Further, officers at the vaccine depot had to be knowledgeable about animal health and hygiene because they had to be competent enough to regulate the daily animal care regimen. This was important, given that operations on calves to cultivate lymph involved a series of preparatory steps, that attention had to be paid to their diet, and sanitary conditions had to be maintained around them. In addition, the physical and psychological trauma undergone by calves during operations concerned the depot. Getting into a collaboration with the Civil Veterinary Department took time and, in the interim, the vaccine depot had to deal with outbreaks of epizootics such as rinderpest, anthrax, and foot-and-mouth disease on its own. The damage done to its finances by these epizootics forced the depot to segregate cattle during outbreaks, and adopt preventive measures such as quarantines and frequent physical examinations in non-epizootic times. Indeed, the vaccine depot's concern for cattle health and disease meant that it usually operated like an animal hospital.

## *Urban and Rural Areas*

An important development in colonial Burma was the emergence of a major gulf between Rangoon, the urban city, and the province's rural areas. The expanding vaccination programme both reflected and contributed to this divide. This study has attempted to show that this spatial and conceptual bifurcation first emerged in what can be called a "medical map". The vaccination establishment found it was operating within the confines of an imagined medical map, defined by the limits of the transportation infrastructure, the vaccine depot, civil hospitals, dispensaries, and towns and villages. This medical map highlighted the division between areas that were easily accessible by road, rivers or rail and areas further out, whose inaccessibility became their defining characteristic in the eyes of the establishment. These were lands in the shadows, where the Vaccination Department could not supervise operations and had to depend on indigenous vaccinators whose returns were considered "untrustworthy". This division was also given textual form in public health reports which began to divide its statistics for each infectious disease, including smallpox, under the heads of "Urban" and "Rural".

The division between urban and rural areas became more pronounced with immigration transforming the urban landscape. The rapid growth of Burma's agricultural economy was sustained by an ever-increasing number of migrant labourers from India, China and Southeast Asia, who together turned Rangoon into a cosmopolitan port city by the turn of the century. Indian immigrants, who formed the majority of the newcomers to Rangoon, lived in unsanitary, crowded lodging houses and became a huge health concern for colonial officers. A tug of war between colonial health officers and members of trade and commerce associations complicated the process of passing laws to make vaccination compulsory for the passengers of incoming vessels. Nevertheless, the addition of large numbers of Indian immigrants to the urban milieu forced the colonial government to treat port cities such as Rangoon differently from other areas of Burma. While other vaccination legislation, such as the Burma Prohibition of Inoculation and Licensing of Vaccinators Act, 1908, was already in place, the colonial authorities passed new laws specifically targeted at immigrants. These included specific regulations those disembarking in Rangoon had to follow, as stipulated in the Burma Vaccination Law Amendment Acts of 1909 and 1928. The limited extension of these Acts into rural areas until the 1920s contributed to, in the eyes of the vaccination establishment, the shadowy image of these remote areas. Though the view of what was accessible and inaccessible fluctuated and changed over the course of the colonial period, there continually remained a "hinterland" in one shape or another that the vaccination establishment could not reach. The colonial government attempted to use the Vaccination Acts to curb the activities of indigenous inoculators who were most active in such rural areas. But these efforts ended in vain because many indigenous inoculators successfully manipulated or otherwise circumvented legislative terminology to evade punishment. Indigenous inoculators survived until the end of colonial rule, leaving a rural Burma largely unconverted by nearly a century of state-enforced vaccination operations.

## *The Rationality of Resistance*

An important obstacle to the extension of vaccination in Burma was indigenous resistance. The medical establishment in British India as a whole viewed it in the context of Hindu society, and attributed it to a range of "irrational" factors. Caste and concern for the well-being of the sacred cow were the most frequently cited factors. Bhattacharya, Harrison, and Worboys have stressed that colonial reports ignored the possibility that Indian resistance could have been rational, a reaction to the unreliability and danger of the vaccination operation. This becomes clear in the case of Burma, for in the absence of caste and veneration of the cow, the indigenous preference for inoculation was due to a rational choice (vaccination was seen to be more dangerous), familiarity (inoculation techniques were similar to those of traditional tattooing) and by default (the limited reach of vaccination could not match the ubiquity of indigenous inoculators).

Some civil surgeons in Burma understood the rational basis of indigenous resistance to vaccination. Rather than blaming superstition, which was the prevailing colonial practice even in this corner of British India, they attributed the lack of interest in vaccination to the failure of the establishment to make a case that was properly understood by the indigenous population. Civil medical officers such as Nisbet felt that the colonial government needed to do much more and circulate "the facts" through Burmese-language treatises. The limited recognition of the rationality of indigenous resistance was an implicit factor in research into better lymph. It was understood early on that bad lymph weakened the case for indigenous acceptance of vaccination. This prodded some colonial medical officers to seek out lymph that would fail and thus suggest that vaccination was a poor choice for smallpox prevention.

The colonial failure to question vaccination or explain it to the Burmese presented a major obstacle to the acceptance of the procedure by the indigenous population. Burmese medical practitioners could have been crucial to popularising vaccination, but the medical establishment failed to mobilise such indigenous agency until later in the colonial period. This failure was partly the result of the colonial medical establishment's refusal to take indigenous medicine seriously until the 1920s. This happened despite several dissenting doctors who tried to convince the Burmese of the efficacy of vaccination and to collaborate with indigenous inoculators. One major contributing factor was that colonial doctors were uncompromising when it came to the superiority of vaccination, spurred on by the unending debates that had taken place in Britain over the safety of vaccination. Another factor was that these doctors viewed Western medicine as scientific and indigenous medicine as unscientific, which made it unworthy of examination. A third factor was that opposition to vaccination was often seen as opposition to their authority, something that had a political motive rather than a medical one. At the same time, the colonial medical establishment was handicapped by some other factors, which probably hindered its ability to understand indigenous medicine, even if it had wanted to. A significant language barrier, poor funding, and understaffing limited its activities, and overburdened doctors had very little time to pay attention to matters outside their immediate responsibilities. All these limitations prevented a fair and comprehensive enquiry into local medical traditions. Indeed, they had very little time to spend even on their own vaccination effort.

# Appendix I

## *Burma Prohibition of Inoculation and Licensing of Vaccinators Act, 1908 (Burma Act 6 of 1908)*[1]

No. *27 A—Dated Rangoon, the 3rd August, 1909.*—With reference to the provisions of section 4, sub-section (1), clause (a) of the Burma Prohibition of Inoculation and Licensing of Vaccinators Act, 1908, the Lieutenant-Governor specifies the following as the medical qualifications which will entitle a person to perform vaccination under this clause:—

(a) A degree of Bachelor of Medicine or Bachelor of Surgery, or any corresponding or higher degree in medicine or surgery granted by a University in Great Britain or India or by any other University, the degrees granted by which the Local Government may accept as of equal value.

(b) A diploma in medicine or surgery or a licence to practise medicine or surgery, granted by a properly constituted examining or licensing body in Great Britain or India, or by any body elsewhere, the licences granted by which the Local Government may accept as of equal value.

No. 275,—*Dated Rangoon, the 3rd August, 1919.*—In exercise of the powers conferred by section 6, sub-section (1) of the Burma Prohibition of Inoculation and Licensing of Vaccinators Act, 1908, the Lieutenant-Governor is pleased to make the following rules to regulate the matters [re]ferred to in that sub-section:—

*Public Vaccinators*

1. No person shall be appointed to be a vaccinator except in accordance with the rules contained in the Civil Service

[1] Issued as an insert in the *Rangoon Municipal Manual* after page 248.

Regulations and such rules as the Local Government may from time to time prescribe to regulate the appointment of persons to Government service.

2. No person shall be appointed to be a vaccinator who is under 18 or over 35 years of age.

3. No person shall be appointed to be a vaccinator who has not passed the Anglo-Vernacular or Vernacular seventh standard examination:

   Provided that persons with a lower educational qualification may in special cases be appointed with the previous sanction of the Superintendent General of Vaccination.

4. No person shall be appointed to be a vaccinator unless he has undergone the training prescribed for public vaccinators from time to time by the Superintendent General of Vaccination, with the approval of the Local Government, and has obtained a certificate from the Superintendent of the Vaccine Depot, Meiktila, that he has attained proficiency in the knowledge and technique required for the preparation of calf lymph.

5. A vaccinator appointed under section 4, sub-section (2) of the Act, may be suspended or dismissed by the officer appointing him in accordance with the rules laid down by the Local Government from time to time for the suspension and dismissal of Government servants.

*Private Vaccinators*

6. No licence shall be granted to any person authorising him to practise vaccination except in accordance with the following conditions:—

   *(a)* the applicant must be over 18 years of age;

   *(b)* the applicant must satisfy the officer granting the licence that he has sufficient technical knowledge to enable him to vaccinate and to treat the persons on whom he operates;

   *(c)* the applicant must, if required, produce a certificate in the following form signed by a qualified medical man :—

   *I do hereby certify that I have examined __________ a candidate for appointment as a private vaccinator, and that I consider that he is physically and mentally fit for appointment. __________'s age is according to his own statement ______________ years and by appearance _________________ years.*

7. All licences issued under section 4, sub-section (2) of the Act, shall be granted in Form I attached to these rules and shall be valid for the area and the period specified therein.

*Suspension and Cancellation of Licences*

8. A licence issued under section 4, sub-section (2) of the Act, may be suspended or cancelled by the officer by whom it was issued, subject to the control of the Superintendent General of Vaccination, if the holder of the licence—
   (a) infringes any of the conditions laid down in Rule 9 below;
   (b) by any action obstructs the proper performance of vaccination by the Government Vaccination Establishment;
   (c) fails to exercise reasonable care in the treatment of any person vaccinated by him;
   (d) demands higher fees than those authorised by the Superintendent General of Vaccination with the approval of the Local Government; or
   (e) does any act which, if he were in Government service, would justify his dismissal therefrom:

   Provided that no licence shall be suspended or cancelled under clause (e) except with the previous approval of the Superintendent General of Vaccination.

9. All persons licensed to practise vaccination as private vaccinators shall comply with the following conditions :—
   (a) The licencee shall observe such regulations as may be published from time to time by the Superintendent General of Vaccination for the performance of vaccination and the treatment of those vaccinated after operation.
   (b) The licencee shall practise vaccination only in the local area in which he is licensed to practise and during the period for which his licence subsists.
   (c) The licencee shall use no lymph that has not been approved by the Superintendent General of Vaccination.

*General Rules for carrying out the purposes of the Act*

10. The Civil Surgeons of all districts, the Health Officer of every Municipality or Port, and any officer specially authorised by the Local Government under the provisions of section 4, sub-section (2), shall maintain a register of licences granted to

private vaccinators in the form shown in Form II attached to these rules,

*FORM I*

*Form of Licence*

I, the undersigned, hereby licence son of __________ residing at ________, who is qualified to act as a private vaccinator under the rules made under section 6 of the Burma Prohibition of Inoculation and Licensing of Vaccinators Act, 1908, to practise vaccination within the limits of the _________ District.

Municipality

Port

Township

for a period of ____ months, commencing from _______ 19___

(Signed)

*Civil Surgeon*

*Health Officer*

*Dated at*

*This ____________ day of _________ 19___*

*Specially authorised by the Local Government.*

*FORM II.*

*Register of Licences*

| Serial number of licence | Date of issue of licence | Name of licence-holder with particulars of residence | Father's name and residence, if alive. | Qualifications, Educational and Technical | The Township or local area within which licence is valid | Period covered by the licence |
|---|---|---|---|---|---|---|
| | | | | | | |

*(Burma Gazette, dated 7th August 1909)*, Part I, page 606.

# *Appendix II*

## *A. Callaway Nisbet's 1869 Treatise on Vaccination*

The Civil Surgeon of Bassein is sorry to find that Burman parents are, as a rule, opposed to Vaccination, which they erroneously look up as the 'Foreigners' Small-Pox,' and that they neglect therefore to avail themselves of means (placed by Government at great expense within their reach) for preventing, and doing away with that horrible disease. Knowing that this arises from ignorance upon the subject, he wishes to say a few words to them, hoping to help those who have no opportunities of learning the truth about it to realise and see the importance of the matter. Every one knows that when a person is inoculated in the Burman fashion he incurs the risk of dying from small-pox, brought on by the operation. Every one who comes near to him, is liable to take the disease, and to spread it in his turn. In short small-pox is thus voluntarily produced and involuntarily propagated; and in this consists the great evil of the system, as epidemics not unfrequently originate in this way, as was the case here in 1867, destroying thousands, depriving them of sight, or disfiguring them for life. Now, the first truth I have to tell about vaccination is, that it never does this. It *never causes* small-pox *kyauk-ma-pauk-wei* [original term in Burmese script]. What is *does* cause, is a harmless pock which never kills, blinds or disfigures. No one I think ever heard (out of Bassein) of vaccination *causing* small-pox. Its worst enemies (for like everything good in this world, it has enemies even among those who might know better) have never accused it of this. Small-pox may, and often does follow after vaccination during epidemics, when vaccination is comparatively inert. But any one observing its effect with any attention, when small-pox is not 'about' may satisfy himself, that the Native belief in its *causing* small-pox is groundless, except they choose to make no distinction between a disease which kills with notorious virulence, and one that only causes some small sores and scars on the arms, which is stupid and absurd. Inoculation then, whatever may be its advantages, produces (as every one knows) small-pox, mildly often and even generally, but still unmistakably small-pox. Vaccination (as every one *may* know if he chooses) does not. This very important point being settled, the next question is: Which is the best protector against the disease? Inoculation which keeps up the supply and propagates the contagion, never suffering it to die out, or vaccination which, as I will now attempt to show, destroys it? No one disputes that inoculation protects from future attacks of small-pox, the individual upon whom it is practiced as well, if not better than vaccination does. But this is done at the risk of his life and the lives of others. Now what has vaccination done in this way? Admitting as every one must, that no risk of this kind is incurred: What is its value as a preventive? The answer is—vaccination prevents small-pox altogether. Not only one, but all are saved by it when properly performed, and strictly carried out. Take the history of the operation in Prussia, and throughout Germany, North and South. There the operation is enforced by law, and has been for nearly half a century. And what has been the result? It may be told in three words. Small-pox is extinct. Medical teachers there are in the habit of speaking to their pupils about it, as a disease previously very fatal and loathsome, now unknown. This is prevention, and something more. It is extinction. Here is another example of its power as a safeguard, under a different set of circumstances. In the Small-pox Hospitals in various parts of Europe, where the disease is not yet stamped out in this energetic way, the preventive power of vaccination is displayed in a very marked way. In those ghastly abodes of suffering humanity, vaccination of the hospital attendants is as strictly carried out, as it is in Prussia, from a different cause, viz, from their natural fear of contagion. The result is, that not a single death from small-pox has been recorded for the last 20 years amongst those thus habitually exposed to the contagion. But some may say vaccination has already been tried here and has failed. And this is, to a great extent true. In 1867 the failures were numerous. The operation naturally got a bad name. Why it failed then is easily explained. The poison of small-pox filled the air and contaminated everything and everybody. Inoculators were busy at work propagating it. The very Vaccinators had it in and around their homes; and still, not wickedly, but ignorantly plied diligently their vocation in rivalry with the Native Inoculators. Nay, the lymph itself was poisoned, but the simultaneous efforts of both upon not a few of the patients, who figure in the records, as successfully vaccinated! Need any more be said? The wonder only is, that even under such circumstances, some 1000 people appear to have benefitted to some extent by operations so conducted, the characters of which did not transpire till it was too late. It follows from what has been said, that to be successful, vaccination must be strictly carried out. And enough has been said I think to show that it is harmless, and that it only requires a fair trial to convince any unbiased observer as to its value as a safeguard against one of the most loathsome diseases which 'flesh is heir to.' But the season for operating in this part of the world is short, and is already nearly over. No time therefore is to be lost, if this healthy season is to be taken advantage of. No one can say how soon small-pox may appear or be imported from abroad, starting the inoculators, and perhaps another epidemic, as in 1867. There are hundreds of unprotected children who have been born here since that visitation. To the parents of these, these words are especially addressed, and most earnestly recommended to their deliberate attention.[2]

[2] *Report on Vaccination for 1868*, appendix, xvi–xviii. Note: Also provided as "Appendix to Bassein Health Report [Treatise on Vaccination and Inoculation]," in *RPHVS for 1868*, 195–97.

# *Bibliography*


PRIMARY SOURCES

**Archival Documents**

*India Office Library, London*

IOR/F/4/11883, Report of the Superintendent General of Vaccination for the Year 1813. "The exertions of Mr. Carey, a missionary and others favourably noticed". Extract from the Public Letter from Bengal, Calcutta, 27 July 1814.

IOR/P/5798 File no. 3Z-32, from His Excellency the Governor-General of India in Council to Her Majesty's Secretary of State for India. No. 33 (Sanitary), Calcutta, 29 December 1898.

IOR/P/5798, from A. D. Warren, Secretary to the Rangoon Chamber of Commerce, to the Secretary to the Government of Burma, 20 June 1899.

IOR/P/5798, notes by Dr J. C. Hoyle, Municipal Health Officer, Rangoon, dated 19 July1899, on the recent Smallpox Epidemic, 1898–99.

IOR/P/5798, from Colonel D. Sinclair, Sanitary Commissioner, Burma, to the Secretary to the Government of Burma, 30 August 1899.

IOR/P/5798, from Commander H. S. Black, Port Officer, Rangoon, to the Secretary to the Government of Burma, 7 October 1899.

IOR/P/5798, from Civil Surgeon and Port Health Officer, Maulmain, to the Deputy Commissioner, Amherst (Sanitary), 6 November 1899.

IOR/P/5798, "Bill to make further provision for compulsory Vaccination in Burma". Legislative Department-No. 1150-1Z-2. From the Secretary to the Government of Burma to the Secretary to the Government of India, Legislative Department, 30 March 1900.

IOR/P/6034 File No. 1Z-5, Colonel C. C. Little, to the Secretary to the Government of Burma, 12 January 1901, Home (Sanitary) Department, Burma, February 1901.

IOR/P/6034, File No. 2T-27, Note by Mr D. Norton, CSI, and Mr C. R. T. Balston on the reorganisation of Municipal establishment in Rangoon, Home (Medical), April 1901.

IOR/P/6034 File no. 1Z-5, Government Order, Rangoon, dated 31 May 1901.

IOR/P/7786 Burma File 1908, P. W. Monie to the Secretary to the Government of Burma, 23 May 1908, Home (Medical) Department, Burma, January 1908.

IOR/P/7786 Burma File 1908, Major J. Entrican to Superintendent of Vaccination, Burma, 15 September 1907, Home (Medical) Department, Burma, January 1908.

IOR/P/7786 Burma File 1908, D. Sherame to the Secretary to the Government of India, 23 January 1908; Colonel King to the Secretary to the Government of Burma, 8 October 1907, Home (Medical) Department, Burma, January 1908.

IOR/P/7791, File no. 2Z-5, Pt. I, no. 1124-2Z-5, from D. Shearme, Esq., ICS, Secretary to the Government of Burma, to the Sanitary Commissioner, Burma, dated 25 March 1908.

IOR/P/7791, File no. 2Z-5, Pt. I, no. 2469-2V.R., from Major C. E. Williams, MD, DPH, IMS, Sanitary Commissioner, Burma, to the Secretary to the Government of Burma, dated 11 April 1908.

IOR/P/7791, File no. 2Z-5, Pt. II, no. 571-4P-3, from M. Laurie, Esq., MVO, ICS, President, Rangoon Municipal Committee, to the Secretary to the Government of Burma, dated 3 July 1908.

IOR/P/7791, File no. 2Z-5, Pt. II, no. 306-2Z-5, from D. Shearme, Esq., ICS, Secretary to the Government of Burma, to the President, Rangoon Municipal Committee, dated 8 August 1908.

IOR/P/7796, Burma File, 1908, Colonel W. G. King to the Secretary to the Government of Burma, 10 January 1908, in Home (Medical) Department, Burma, January 1908.

IOR/L/PJ/6/640 File 1413, J. B. Wingate to the Secretary to the Government of India, Home Department, 27 February 1903, Judicial and Public Papers (1903).

IOR/V/24/4409, V.2., 1891–92 to 1907–8, Annual Report of the Civil Veterinary Department, Burma for the year ending 31st March 1900.

*National Archives of the Union of Myanmar, Yangon*

1/1 (A) Accession no. 97, 1854, File 40, "Introduction of Vaccination into Pegu", 2pp., Box 1854 (3). Colonel Arthur Phayre to the Secretary to the Government of India, Foreign Department, Rangoon, dated 10 November 1854.

1/1 (A) Accession no. 322, 1857, File 51, "Memorial of Dr Dawson on Behalf of the American Baptist Mission for the Exemption of Land and Houses from Usual Taxes in Rangoon", 3pp., Box 1857 (3).

1/1 (A) Accession no. 399, 1858, File 73, "Examination of Medical Officers in Colloquial Burmese", 16pp., Box 1858 (3). Letter to the Secretary to the Government of India, Foreign Department, dated Rangoon, 28 June 1858.

1/1 (A) Accession no. 399, 1858, File 73, "Examination of Medical Officers in Colloquial Burmese", 16pp., Box 1858 (3). Letter from R. B. Chapman,

Esquire, Officiating Undersecretary to the Government of India, to Major Arthur Phayre, Commisioner of Pegue, dated 6 August 1858.

1/1 (A) Accession no. 399, 1858, File 73, "Examination of Medical Officers in Colloquial Burmese in Pegu", 16pp., Box 1858 (3). Attachment to Phayre, Letter to Cecil Beadon, Secretaty to the Government of India, Officer to Foreign Department, Fort William, dated Rangoon, 25 August 1858.

1/1 (A) Accession no. 399, 1858, File 73, "Examination of Medical Officers in Colloquial Burmese in Pegu", 16pp., Box 1858 (3). Letter to [Cecil Beaden] the Secretary to the Government of India, Officiating in the Foreign Department, Fort William, dated Rangoon, 31 August 1858.

1/1(A) 1032, 1867, 425, "Mr Dawson's Refusal to Pay Night Watch Tax in Maulmain", Box 1867 (9). Letter from R. Macrae, Maulmain, to Colonel D. Brown, Commissioner of Tenasserim Division, dated Maulmain, 10 August 1867.

1/1 (A) Accession 609, 1863, File no. 45, 6pp., "Extension of Vaccination in British Burma", Box 1863 (2). Letter from Captain H. Nelson Davies, Secretary to the Chief Commissioner of British Burma, and Agent to the Governor General, to Colonel H. M. Durand CB, Secretary to the Governor of India, Foreign Department, Governor General's Headquarters at Calcutta, dated Rangoon, 2 May 1863.

1/1(A) Accession 612, 1863, 49 "Apptt. Of Asstt. Surgeon A. J. Cowie as Civil Surgeon at Rangoon in the Room of Asstt. Surgeon J. E. Dickenson resigned". 12pp. Box 1863 (2). Letter from Davies, Secretary to Chief Commissioner, British Burma and Agent to Colonel Durand, dated Rangoon, 6 January 1863.

1/1(A) Accession 612, 1863, 49 "Apptt. Of Asstt. Surgeon A. J. Cowie as Civil Surgeon at Rangoon in the Room of Asstt. Surgeon J. E. Dickenson resigned". 12pp. Box 1863 (2). Letter from Davies, Secretary to Chief Commissioner, British Burma to the Officiating Secretary to the Government of India, dated Rangoon, 9 July 1863.

1/1 (A) Accession 614, 1863, File no. 43, 14pp., "Grant of Leave to Dr. J. Davis, Surgeon of Bassein", Box 1863 (2). Letter from the Secretary to the Governor General of India to Chief Commissioner, British Burma, dated Simla, 26 June 1863.

1/1 (A) Accession 778, 1866, File no. 237, "Public Health", 18pp., Box 1866 (4). Minute by the Chief Commissioner of British Burma, dated Camp at Pounglay, district of Prome, 27 February 1866.

1/1(A) Accession 859, 1867, File no. 70, 8pp., Box 1867(3). W. A. Green, Memorandum, to the Secretary to the Government of India, in the Home Department, no. 1748B, dated 5 February 1867.

1/1(A) Accession 1083, 1867–68, 5 (2) "Treatise on Vaccination in the Vernacular", 72 pp., Box 1868 (1). Letter from A. C. Nisbet, Superintendent, Bassein Jail, to Charles Planck, Inspector General of Prisons, dated Bassein, 20 December 1867.

1/1 (A) Accession 1083, 1867–68, File no. 5 (2) "Treatise on Vaccination in the Vernacular", 72pp. Box 1868 (1). Letter from Colonel D. Brown, Commissioner of Tenasserim Division, British Burma, to the Horace Spearman, Esquire, Officiating Assistant Secretary to the Chief Commissioner, dated 4 February 1868.

1/1 (A) Accession 1083, 1867–68, File no. 5 (2) "Treatise on Vaccination in the Vernacular" 72pp. Box 1868 (1). Letter from Dr. W. Miller, Civil Surgeon, Thayet-myo, to Commissioner of Pegu, dated Rangoon, 21 February 1868.

1/1 (A) Accession 1083, 1867–68, File no. 5 (2) "Treatise on Vaccination in the Vernacular" 72pp. Box 1868 (1). Letter from the Deputy Commissioner of Tavoy to the Commissioner at Maulmain, dated 4 March 1868.

1/1 (A) Accession 1083, 1867–68, File no. 5 (2) "Treatise on Vaccination in the Vernacular", 72pp. Box 1868 (1). Letter from Charles Planck, Inspector General of Prison, British Burma, to Horace Spearman, Esquire, Assistant Secretary to the Chief Commissioner, dated Rangoon, 2 April 1868.

1/1 (A) Accession 1374, 1867–68, File no. 442 "Mason's Materia Medica". 31pp. Box 1868 (19). Letter from Horace Spearman, Officiating Secretary to Captain C. D. Hildebrand, Officiating Secretary to the Chief Commissioner, British Burma, to the Secretary to the Government of India, Home Department, dated Rangoon, 20 February 1867.

1/15 (C), Accession 290, 1924, File 3M-13, "Proposal for Opening Training *Sesayas* in Western Medicine at Bassein", 18pp., Box 10. Letter from Colonel P. Dee, MB, IMS, Inspector General of Civil Hospitals, Burma, to Commissioner, Irawaddy Division, Bassein, dated Rangoon, 16 June 1924.

1/15 (C), Accession 290, 1924, File 3M-13, "Proposal for Opening Training *Sesayas* in Western Medicine at Bassein", 18pp., Box 10. Major W. L. Brooks, IMD, Civil Surgeon, Myaungmya, "List of Burmese *Saysayas* who are willing to undergo training in Western Medicine at Bassein", attached to letter to the Deputy Commissioner, Myaungmya, dated 2 September 1924.

**Official Reports and Publications**

"Abstract of the Proceedings of the Council of the Lieutenant-Governor of Burma".

*Administration Report*. For 1868–69 to 1870–71. Rangoon: Chief Commissioner's Office Press; Secretariat Press.

*Annual Report of the Health Officer for the City of Rangoon for the year 1927*. Rangoon: The Burma Guardian Press, 1927.

*Annual Report of the Medical Department for the Year 1931 (Federated Malay States)*. Kuala Lumpur: Federated Malay States Government Printing Office, 1932.

*Annual Report of the Public Health Commissioner with the Government of India.* For the Years 1925 to 1936. Calcutta: Government of India Central Publication Branch.

"Annual Report on the Working of the Taunggyi Vaccine Depot for 1899–1900". In *Notes and Statistics on Vaccination in Burma for 1899–1900*, Appendix B.

*The Burma Hand-Book of Rural Self Government*. 2 vols. Rangoon: Office of the Superintendent, Government Printing and Stationery, Union of Burma, 1957.

*Notes and Statistics on Hospitals and Dispensaries in Burma for the Year 1917*. Rangoon: Office of the Superintendent, Government Printing, Burma, 1918.

*Notes and Statistics on Hospitals and Dispensaries in Burma*. For the Years 1917 to 1918. Rangoon: Office of the Superintendent, Government Printing, Burma.

*Notes and Statistics on Vaccination in Burma*. For the Years 1894–95 to 1921–22. Rangoon: Office of the Superintendent, Government Printing, Burma.

*Rangoon Municipality Handbook*. 6th edition. Rangoon: Office of the Superintendent, Government Printing, Burma, 1908.

*Report of the Committee of Enquiry into the Indigenous System of Medicine*. Rangoon: Office of the Superintendent, Government Printing and Stationery, Burma, 1951.

*Report of the Medical Officer*, supplement to *Annual Report of the Local Government Board*. For the Years 1876, 1878–79 to 1882–83, 1883 to 1890, 1891–92 to 1904–5. London: George E. Eyre and William Spottiswoode.

*Report on Public Health and Vital Statistics in British Burma*. For the Years 1867 to 1869. Rangoon: Chief Commissioner's Press, 1870.

*Report on Public Instruction in British Burma*. For the Years 1872–73 to 1893–94. Rangoon: Government Printing Press.

*Report on Sanitary Measures in India*. For 1874–75 to 1907–08. London: HMSO.

*Report on the Administration of British Burma*. For the Years 1872–73 to 1884–85. Rangoon: Government Press.

*Report on the Administration of Burma*. For the Years 1888–89 to 1933–36. Rangoon: Government Printing and Stationery.

*Report on the Administration of Lower Burma during 1885–86 and on the Administration of Upper Burma during 1886*. Rangoon: Superintendent, Government Printing, Burma, 1887.

*Report on the Administration of Lower Burma during 1886–87*. Rangoon: Superintendent, Government Printing and Stationery, Burma, 1888.

*Report on the Administration of Province of British Burma*. For the Years 1861–62 to 1869–70. Rangoon: Military Orphan Press; Foreign Department Press; Central Gaol Press.

*Report on the Administration of the Province of Pegu*. For the Years 1855–56 to 1860–61. Rangoon. N.p.

*Report on the Health of the Indigenous Peoples of British Burma, and on the Supposed Causes of the Sparseness of the Population in that Province*. Rangoon: Rangoon Times Press, 1864.

*Report on the Public Health Administration of Burma*. For the Years 1929–39. Rangoon: Superintendent of Government Printing and Stationery, Burma.

*Report on the State of Public Health in Burma during 1938*. Rangoon: Superintendent, Government Printing and Stationery, Burma, 1939.

*Report on Vaccination for 1867–68*. Rangoon: Rangoon Times Press, 1868.

*Report on Vaccination for 1868*. Maulmain: Advertiser Press, 1870.

*Report on Vaccination in British Burma for the year 1869–70*. Rangoon: Central Gaol Press, 1870.

*Report on Vaccination in Burma*. During the Years 1870–71 to 1871–72. Rangoon: British Burma Press; for the Years 1889–90 to 1893–94. Rangoon: Government Printing.

*A Reprint of the Printed Judgments of the Court of the Judicial Commissioner, Lower Burma, and the Special Court For the Period extended from 1893–1900*. Rangoon: Superintendent, Government Printing, 1902.

*Selected Correspondence and Letters for the Years 1825–26 to 1842–43 in the Office of the Commissioner Tenasserim Division*. Rangoon: Office of the Superintendent, Government Printing, Burma, 1929.

*Triennial Report on Vaccination in Burma*. For the Years 1890–91, 1891 92, and 1892–93 to 1917–18, 1918–19, and 1919–20. Rangoon: Office of the Superintendent, Government Printing, Burma.

*The Upper Burma Rulings 1897–1901. Criminal. Volume I*. Rangoon: Superintendent, Government Printing and Stationery, Burma, 1931.

Wehinger, Father S. J., comp. *Report on St. John's Leper Asylum, Mandalay, Upper Burma, For the Year 1902–3*. Rangoon: Office of the Superintendent, Government Printing, Burma, 1903.

### Contemporary Newspapers and Journals

"Burma Branch". *Supplement to the British Medical Journal* (30 April 1910), 189–95.

"The Burma Government Resolution on Indigenous Medicine". *Indian Medical Gazette* 63 (April, 1928), 205–6.

"Burma Legislative Council", *Rangoon Times* (Saturday, 29 August 1908).

Eugenio Kincaid to Dr. L. Bolles, dated Ava, 15 February 1834, *American Baptist Missionary Magazine* 15 no. 1, 1835, 39.

"Extracts of Letters from Rev. A Judson to Rev. G.H. Hough Now at Serampore. January 22, 1821", *American Baptist Missionary Magazine* 3.7 (1822), 256.

Judson, Adoniram. "Extracts of Letters from Rev. A Judson to Rev. G.H. Hough Now at Serampore. January 22, 1821". *American Baptist Missionary Magazine* 3.7 (1822), 256.

Letter from John Taylor Jones to the Reverend L. Bolles, 30 May 1833, Bangkok, in *American Baptist Missionary Magazine* 16.6 (1836), 300.

*London Times*

*Maulmain Chronicle* (18 November 1837), 127.

*Maulmain Chronicle* (26 January 1842).

*Rangoon Gazette and Weekly Budget* (18 July 1890).

*Rangoon Gazette and Weekly Budget* (26 June 1896), 11.
*Rangoon Gazette and Weekly Budget* (21 August 1896).
*Rangoon Gazette and Weekly Budget* (26 September 1896).
*Rangoon Gazette and Weekly Budget* (21 November 1896), 4.
*Rangoon Gazette and Weekly Budget* (24 April 1897), 29.
*Rangoon Gazette and Weekly Budget* (29 May 1899), 15–16.
"Surgery in Burmah". *British Medical Journal* 2 (23 October 1886), 1063.
*Times of Burma* (22 July 1905), 5.
*Times of Burma* (9 September 1905), 5.
*Times of Burma* (27 January 1906), 6.
*Times of Burma* (3 March 1906), 5–6.
*Times of Burma* (24 February 1906), 12.
*Times of Burma* (3 March 1906), 6.
*Times of Burma* (17 March 1906), 12.
"Upper Burma". *British Medical Journal* 2 (November, 1886), 1062.
"Vaccination in British Burma". *British Medical Journal* 1 (27 May 1882), 791.
"Vaccination in Burma". *Rangoon Gazette Weekly Budget* (18 July 1890).
"Vaccination in Burma". *British Medical Journal* 1 (5 March 1894), 499.
"Vaccination in Burma". *British Medical Journal* 1 (2 April 1898), 927–28._

**Books**

Alcott, William A. *The House I Live in; or the Human Body*. 3rd ed. Rangoon: American Missions Press, 1875.

Andrus, J. Russell. *Rural Reconstruction in Burma*. London: Oxford University Press, n.d.

Balfour, Edward. *The Cyclopædia of India and of Eastern and Southern Asia, Commercial, Industrial, and Scientific; Products of the Mineral, Vegetable and Animal Kingdom, Useful Arts and Manufactures*. 3 vols. 3rd ed. London: Bernard Quaritch, 1885.

Bastian, Adolf. *A Journey in Burma (1861–1862)*. Bangkok: White Lotus, 2004.

Brown, Thomas. *An Investigation of the Present Unsatisfactory and Defective State of Vaccination; and the Several Expedients Proposed for Removing the Now Acknowledged Defects of the Jennerian Practice*. Edinburgh: Maclachlan, Stewart & Co, 1842.

Bryce, James. *Practical Observations on the Inoculation of Cowpox*. Edinburgh, 1802.

*Burma Gazetteer: Tharrawaddy District*. Vol. A. Rangoon: Superintendent, Government Printing and Stationery, Union of Burma, 1959.

Castor, R. H. *Nomenclature of Diseases in Burmese*. Rangoon: Superintendent, Government Printing, Burma, 1922.

Colbeck, James Alfred. *Letters from Mandalay: A Series of Letters by the late James Alfred Colbeck*. London: Alfred W. Lowe, 1882.

Cullimore, Daniel Henry. *Medical History of the People of India: The Burmese, What do They Know of Medicine?* Madras: Higginbotham, 1875.

Entrican, J. *Notes for the Use of Vaccinators*. Rangoon: Government Press, 1918.

Fujikawa, Yu. *Nihon Sippei-shi*. Tokyo: Heibonsha, 1869.

Grant Brown, R. *Burma as I Saw It, 1889–1917: With a Chapter on Recent Events*. London: Methuen, 1926.

Halliday, Robert. *The Talaings*. Rangoon: Superintendent, Government Printing, Burma, 1917.

Hamilton, Alexander. *A New Account of the East Indies*, 2 vols. London: Argonaut Press, 1930.

Hardiman, J. P., comp. *Burma Gazeteer: Lower Chindwin District*. Rangoon: Central Press, 1967.

*The History of Inoculation and Vaccination for the Prevention and Treatment of Disease*. Lecture Memoranda. XVIIth International Congress of Medicine, London. London: Burroughs Wellcome, 1913.

*Hman-nan maha-ya-zawin-daw-gyi*. Vol. 1. Yangon, 1967.

Ito, Sakae. *Ito Genboku-den*. Tokyo: Genbun-sha, 1916.

Jenner, Edward. *An Inquiry into the Causes and Effects of the Variolæ Vaccine, A Disease Discovered in Some of the Western Counties of England, Particularly Gloucestershire, and Known by the Name of The Cow Pox*. London: Sampson Low, 1798.

King, W. G. *Vaccination in the Tropics*. London: Tropical Diseases Bureau, 1920.

MacDonald, Keith Norman. *The Practice of Medicine Among the Burmese. Translated from Original Manuscripts with an Historical Sketch of the Progress of Medicine from the Earliest Times*. Edinburgh: MacLachlan and Stewart, 1879.

McVail, John C. *Half a Century of Smallpox and Vaccination*. Edinburgh: E. and S. Livingston, 1919.

Malcom, Howard. *Travels in South-Eastern Asia, Embracing Hindustan, Malaya, Siam, and China; With Notices of Numerous Missionary Stations, and a Full Account of the Burman Empire*. 2 vols. 2nd ed. Boston: Gould, Kendall, and Lincoln, 1839.

——. *Travels in the Burman Empire*. Bangkok: Ava House, 1997.

Mason, Rev. *A Burmese Hand-book of Medicine. Ingalei-hseì-kyan*. Toungoo: Karen Institute Press, 1866.

Nisbet, John. *Burma under British Rule—and Before*. 2 vols. Westminster: Archibald Constable & Co, 1901.

Pearce, Charles T. M.D. *Vaccination: Its Tested Effects on Health, Mortality, and Population*. London: H. Baillier Brothers, 1868.

Sangermano, Vicenzo. *Description of the Burmese Empire*. Translated by William Tandy. Rome: Oriental Translation Fund of Great Britain and Ireland, 1833.

Searle, H. F., comp. *Burma Gazetteer: The Mandalay District*. Rangoon: Superintendent of Government Printing and Stationery, 1928.

Shway Yoe [James George Scott]. *The Burman His Life and Notions*. London: MacMillan, 1910.

Spinzig, C. Variola: Its Causes, Nature and Prophylaxis, and the Dangers of Vaccination. St. Louis, Missouri: Buxton and Skinner, 1878.

Stewart, J. A. *Kyaukse Gazetteer*. Rangoon, 1925.

Tin, U. (Mandalay), comp. *Kon-baung-zet-maha-ya-zawin-daw-gyi*. 3 vols. Rangoon: Leidi Mangain, 1967.

Tout, *hsaya. Ingalei-hseì-kyan*. Rangoon: Bengalee Job Printing Press, 1881.

*Variola and Vaccinia: History and Description*. Boston: New England Vaccine Company, n.d.

*Who's Who in Burma: A Biographical Record of Prominent Residents of Burma*. Calcutta and Rangoon: Indo-Burma Publishing Agency, 1926.

**Articles in Journals and Transactions**

Castor, R. H. "Inoculation, Vaccination and Smallpox". *Journal of Tropical Medicine and Hygiene* 15, no. 18, 1912, 278–81.

Copeman, S. Monckton. "The Inter-relationship of Variola and Vaccinia". *Proceedings of the Royal Society of London* 71, 1902–3, 121–33.

Cunningham, J., and J. A. Cruickshank. "An Investigation into the Relative Values of Lanoline and Glycerine as Vehicles for Vaccine Lymph in the Tropics". *Indian Journal of Medical Research* 11, 1923–24, 1173–203.

Entrican, J. "A Civil Surgeon 'on Tour' in Upper Burma". *Indian Medical Gazette* 54, no. 1, 1919, 1–9.

Green, Alan B. "Preliminary Notes on the Use of Chloroform in the Preparation of Vaccine". *Proceedings of the Royal Society of London* 72, 1903–4, 1–4.

——. "Further Note on Some Additional Points in Connection with Chloroformed Calf Vaccine". *Proceedings of the Royal Society of London* 73, 1904, 342–46.

Greenwood, M. "The Vaccination Problem". *Journal of the Royal Statistical Society* 93, no. 2 , 1930, 233–70.

Harvey, W. F. "Vaccine Lymphs in the Punjab". *Indian Medical Gazette* 40, no. 3, 1905, 85–90.

——. "Vaccine Lymph Production, Preparation, and Preservation". *Indian Journal of Medical Research* 8, 1920–21, 257–69.

Highet, H. Campbell. "Small Pox, Vaccination and the New Vaccination Law in Siam". *Journal of the Siam Society* 11, no. 1, 1914–15, 13–25.

Iyer, S. Rama. "Generalized Vaccinia in Burma". *Indian Medical Gazette* 54, 1919, 459–60.

Kinyoun, J. J. "The Action of Glycerin on Bacteria in the Presence of Cell Exudates". *Journal of Experimental Medicine* 7, no. 6, 1905, 725–32.

Mason, Rev. V. "The Liquidamber Tree of the Tenasserim Provinces". *Journal of the Asiatic Society of Bengal* 17, 1848, 532–33.

Nijland, A. N. "Jahresbericht der Kuhpockenanstalt und des Instituts Pasteur in Weltevreden (Java) über das Jahr 1912". *Janus* 18, 1913, 543–57.

Noguchi, Hideyo. "Pure Cultivation in Vivo of Vaccine Virus Free from Bacteria". *Journal of Experimental Medicine* 21, 1915, 539–70.

Pearn, B. R. "Felix Carey and the English Baptist Mission to Burma". *Journal of Burma Research Society* 28, 1938, 12–13.

Reed, Walter. "On the Appearance of Certain Amoeboid Bodies in the Blood of Vaccinated Monkeys (Rhoesus) and Children, in the Blood from Cases of Variola". *Journal of Experimental Medicine* 2, 1897, 515–27.

Sein Khwe, U. "Kyauk yoga: kagwe-ye hnin kudanyi" [Smallpox: Prevention and Treatement]. In *Thudaw ye daw myanma hse pinya* (Yangon: Pyidu kyanma-ye akyawpyu, n.d.), 3: 33–44.

Simpson, W. J. "Observations on the Etiology of Vaccinia and on the Cultivation of the Microbe of Variola". *Journal of Tropical Medicine and Hygiene* 15, no. 14, 15 July 1912, 209–11.

SECONDARY SOURCES

**Books**

Arnold, David. *Colonizing the Body: State Medicine and Epidemic Disease in Nineteenth-Century India*. Berkeley: University of California Press, 1993.

Bala, Poonam. *Imperialism and Medicine in Bengal*. New Delhi: Sage Publications, 1991.

Baldwin, Peter. *Contagion and the State in Europe, 1830–1930*. Cambridge: Cambridge University Press, 2005.

Ban, Tadayasu. *Tekijyuku to Nagayo Sensai: Eiseigaku to Shokakoshi*. Osaka: Sogensha, 1987.

Bayly, C. A. *Empire and Information: Intelligence Gathering and Social Communication in India, 1780–1870*. Cambridge: Cambridge University Press, 1996.

Bevoise, Ken de. *Agents of Apocalypse: Epidemic Disease in the Colonial Philippines*. Princeton, New Jersey: Princeton University Press, 1995.

Bhattacharya, Sanjoy, Mark Harrison, and Michael Worboys. *Fractured States: Smallpox, Public Health and Vaccination Policy in British India, 1800–1947*. London: Sangam Books Limited, 2005.

Bower, John Z. *Medical Education in Japan: From Chinese Medicine, to Western Medicine*. New York: Harper & Row, 1965.

Briggs, Laura. *Reproducing Empire: Race, Sex, Science, and U.S. Imperialism in Puerto Rico*. Berkeley: University of California Press, 2002.

Bynum, W. F., and Roy Porter, eds. *Companion Encyclopedia of the History of Medicine*. 2 vols. London and New York: Routledge, 1997.

Cady, John Frank. *A History of Modern Burma*. Ithaca, New York: Cornell University Press, 1958.

Callahan, Mary P. *Making Enemies: War and State Building in Burma*. Ithaca and Singapore: Cornell University Press and Singapore University Press, 2004.

Charney, Michael W. *Powerful Learning: Buddhist Literati and the Throne in Burma's Last Dynasty*. Ann Arbor, Michigan: University of Michigan Centers for South and Southeast Asian Studies. 2006.

Chatterjee, S. *Meeting the Personalities: Burma Series*. Rangoon: n.p., n.d.

Cooper, Frederick, and Ann Laura Stoler, eds., *Tensions of Empire: Colonial Cultures in a Bourgeois World*. Berkeley/Los Angeles/London: University of California Press, 1997.

Cunningham, Andrew, and Bridie Andrews, eds. *Western Medicine as Contested Knowledge*. Manchester and New York: Manchester University Press, 1997.

Dikötter, Frank, Lars Laamann, and Zhou Xun. *Narcotic Culture: A History of Drugs in China*. Chicago: University of Chicago Press, 2004.

Dirckx, John H., ed. *Stedman's Concise Medical Dictionary for the Health Professions*. Illustrated 4th ed. Philadelphia: Lippincott Williams & Wilkins, 2001.

Durbach, Nadja. *Bodily Matters: The Anti-Vaccination Movement in England, 1853–1907*. Durham and London: Duke University Press, 2005.

Foucault, Michel. *Discipline and Punish: The Birth of the Prison*. Translated from the French by Alan Sheridan. New York: Vintage Books, 1979.

Fujikawa, Hideo. *Fujikawa Yu Chosaku-syu 4*. Kyoto: Shibunkaku, 1981.

Fukase, Yasuaki. *Tennento Konzetsu-shi: Kindai Igaku bokko-ki no hitobito*. Kyoto: Shibunkaku, 2002.

Furnivall, J. S. *Colonial Policy and Practice: A Comparative Study of Burma and Netherlands India*. Cambridge: Cambridge University Press, 1948.

——. *The Fashioning of Leviathon: The Beginnings of British Rule in Burma*. Edited by Gehan Wijeyewardene. Canberra: Australian National University, 1991.

Ghosh, Birendra Nath. *A Treatise on Hygiene and Public Health (Preventive and Social Medicine)*, 15th ed. Calcutta: Scientific Publishing Co, 1969.

Harrison, Mark. *Public Health in British India: Anglo-Indian Preventive Medicine 1859–1914*. Cambridge: Cambridge University Press, 1994.

——. *Climates and Constitutions: Health, Race, Environment, and British Imperialism in India, 1600–1850*. Oxford/New York: Oxford University Press, 1999.

Hayne, Douglas M. *Imperial Medicine: Patrick Manson and the Conquest of Tropical Disease*. Philadelphia: University of Pennsylvania Press, 2001.

Headrick, Daniel R. *Tools of Empire: Technology and European Imperialism in the Nineteenth Century*. Oxford: Oxford University Press, 1981.

Hla Maung. *Myanmar Traditional Medicine: Manual for Health Basic Training Course*. State Traditional Medical Council. The Union of Myanmar. n.d.

Hopkins, Donald. *The Greatest Killer: Smallpox in History,* with a New Introduction. Chicago and London: University of Chicago Press, 2002.

Howell, Joel. *Technology in the Hospital: Transforming Patient Care in the Early Twentieth Century*. Baltimore: John Hopkins University Press, 1995.

Hunt, Nancy Rose. *A Colonial Lexicon of Birth Ritual, Medicalization, and Mobility in the Congo*. Durham: Duke University Press, 1999.

Johnston, William. *The Modern Epidemic: A History of Tuberculosis in Japan*. Cambridge: Harvard University Press, 1995.

Kahrs, Robert F. *Viral Diseases of Cattle*. 2nd ed. Ames: Iowa State University Press, 2001.

Kawashima, Masato. *Rangaku no Izumi koko ni waku: Buzen, Nakatsu Igaku-shi Sanpo*. Oita: Nishinihon Rinsho-igaku Kenkyusho, 1996.

Koike, Toichi. *Igai-shi*. Tokyo: Nihon Shoni Iji Syuppan, 2000.

Konishi, Yoshimaro. *Ogata Koan to Osaka Joto-kan*. Osaka: Toho syuppan, 2002.

Kumar, Anil. *Medicine and the Raj: British Medical Policy in India, 1835–1911*. New Delhi: Sage Publications, 1998.

Kumar, Deepak. *Science and the Raj, 1857–1905*. Delhi: Oxford University Press, 1997.

Leslie, Charles, ed. *Asian Medical Systems: A Comparative Study*. Berkeley: University of California Press, 1976.

Lieberman, Victor. *Burmese Administrative Cycle: Anarchy and Conquest, c. 1580–1760*. Princeton: Princeton University Press, 1984.

MacLeod, Roy, and Milton Lewis, eds. *Disease, Medicine, and Empire: Perspectives on Western Medicine and the Experience of European Expansion*. London and New York: Routledge, 1988.

Manderson, Lenore. *Sickness and the State: Health and Illness in Colonial Malaya*. Cambridge: Cambridge University Press, 1996.

Miichi, Masatosi, and Saito, Osamu and Wakimura, Kohei and Iijima, Wataru. eds. *Sippei, Kaihatsu, Teikoku Iryo: Ajia ni okeru Byoki to Iryo no Rekishigaku*. Tokyo: Tokyo Daigaku Syuppan, 2001.

Mrázek, Rudolf. *Engineers of Happy Land: Technology and Nationalism in a Colony*. Princeton and Oxford: Princeton University Press, 2002.

*Myanma Taingyinhsepinya Thamaing* [History of Indigenous Medical Knowledge]. Yangon: Department of Ministry of Health, 1978.

Nash, Manning. *The Golden Road to Modernity; Village Life in Contemporary Burma*. Chicago: University of Chicago Press, 1965.

Onuki, Emiko. *Nihon-jin no Byoki-kan: Shocho Jinruigakuteki Kosatsu*. Tokyo: Iwanami-shoten. n.d.

Osterhammel, Jürgen. *Colonialism: A Theoretical Overview*. Translated from the German by Shelley L. Frisch. Kingston: Ian Randle Publishers, 1997.

Pati, Biswamoy, and Mark Harrison, eds. *Heatlh, Medicine and Empire: Perspectives on Colonial India*. New Delhi: Orient Longman, 2001.

Pond, Caroline M. *The Fats of Life*. Cambridge: Cambridge University Press, 1998.

Razzell, Peter. *The Conquest of Smallpox: The Impact of Inoculation on Smallpox Mortality in Eighteenth-Century Britain*. Sussex: New Haven Press, 1977.

——. *Edward Jenner's Cowpox Vaccine: The History of a Medical Myth*. Sussex: Caliban Books, 1977.

Richell, Judith L. *Disease and Demography in Colonial Burma*. Singapore: National University of Singapore Press, 2006.

Sakai, Shizu. *Yamai ga kataru Nihon-shi*. Tokyo: Kodan-sha, 2002.

Scott, James C. *Seeing Like a State: How Certain Schemes to Improve the Human Condition Have Failed*. New Haven: Yale University Press, 1998.

Shattuck, George Cheevar. *Diseases of the Tropics*. New York: Appleton Century Crofts, 1951.

Shwe Wa, Maung. *Burma Baptist Chronicle*. 2 vols. Rangoon: Board of Publications, Burma Baptist Convention, 1963.

Silanandabhivumsa, Ashin. *The Venerable Mahasi Sayadaw Biography*, abridged ed. Pt. I. Translated by U Mn Swe (Min Kyaw Thu). Rangoon: U Min Swe, 1982.

Soekawa, Masao. "Gyuto Syuto-hou Shorei no Hanga ni tsuite" [Propaganda Bills for Vaccination Distributed duing the Kaei Period in Japan.]. *Nihon Ishigaku Zasshi* 30, no.1, January 1984, 62–84.

Sullivan, Rodney. "Cholera and Colonialism in the Philippines, 1899–1903". In *Disease, Medicine, and Empire: Perspectives on Western Medicine and the Experience of European Expansion*, ed. Roy Macleod and Milton Lewis, 284–300. London: Routledge, 1988.

Tennyson, F. Jesse. *The Story of Burma*. New York: AMS Press, 1975.

Thant Myint-U. *The Making of Modern Burma*. Cambridge: Cambridge University Press, 2001.

*Who's Who in Burma 1961*. Rangoon: People's Literature Committee and House, 1961.

Worboys, Michael. *Spreading Germs: Disease Theories and Medical Practice in Britain, 1865–1900*. Cambridge: Cambridge University Press, 2000.

## Articles in Books and Journals

Arnold, David. "Smallpox and Colonial Medicine in Nineteenth-Century India". In *Imperial Medicine and Indigenous Societies*, ed. David Arnold, 45–65. Manchester: Manchester University Press, 1988.

——. "Introduction: Disease, Medicine and Empire". In *Imperial Medicine and Indigenous Societies*, ed. David Arnold, 1–26. Manchester: Manchester University Press, 1988.

——. "Medicine and Colonialism". In *Companion Encyclopedia of the History of Medicine*, ed. W. F. Bynum and Roy Porter, 2: 1393–1411. London: Routledge, 2001.

Bailkin, Jordanna. "Making Faces: Tattooed Women and Colonial Regimes", *History Workshop Journal* 59, 2005, 33–56.

Beukers, Harmen. "Mohnike and Vaccination: Deshima-Doctor in the Wake of Von Siebold". *Nihon Ishigaku Zasshi* 48, no.1, 2002, 131–52.

——. "The Fight Against Smallpox in Japan: The Value of Western Medicine Proved". In *Red-Hair Medicine: Dutch-Japanese Medical*

*Relations*, ed. H. Beukers, A. M. Luyendijk-Elkshout, M. E. van Opstall, and F. Vos, 59–77. Amsterdam: Rodopi, 1991.

Bhattacharya, Sanjoy. "Re-devising Jennerian Vaccine?" In *Health, Medicine, and Empire: Perspectives on Colonial India*, ed. Biswamoy Pati and Mark Harrison, 217–69. New Delhi: Orient Longman, 2001.

Boomgaard, Peter. "Smallpox and Vaccination on Java, 1780–1860: Medical Data as a Source for Demographic History". In *Dutch Medicine in the Malay Archipelago, 1816–1942*, ed. A. M. Luyendijk-Elshout, G. M. van Heteren, A. de Knecht-van Eekelen, and M. J. D. Poulissen, 119–31. Amsterdam: Rodopi, 1989.

——. "Smallpox, Vaccination, and the Pax Neerlandica Indonesia, 1550–1930". *Bijdragen tot de Taal-, Land- en Volkenkunde* 159, no. 4, 2003, 590–617.

——. "The Development of Colonial Health Care in Java: An Exploratory Introduction". *Bijdragen tot de Taal-, Land- en Volkenkunde* 149, 1993, 77–93.

Brimnes, Niels. "Variolation, Vaccination and Popular Resistance in Early Colonial South India". *Medical History* 48, 2004, 199–228.

Collier, L. H. "The Preservation of Vaccinia Virus". *Microbiology and Molecular Biology Reviews* 18 (1954), 74–86.

Durbach, Nadja. "'They Might As Brand Us': Working-Class Resistance to Vaccination in Victoria England". *The Society for the Social History of Medicine* 13, no. 1, April 2000, 44–62.

——. "Class, Gender, and the Conscientious Objector to Vaccination, 1898–1907". *Journal of British Studies* 41, no.1, January 2002, 58–83.

Ernst, Waltraud. "Plural Medicine, Tradition and Modernity: Historical and Contemporary Perspectives: Views from Below and From Above". In *Plural Medicine, Tradition and Modernity, 1800–2000*, ed. Waltraud Ernst, 1–19. London: Routledge, 2002.

Fitzgerald, Rosemary. "'Clinical Christianity': The Emergence of Medical Work as a Missionary Strategy in Colonial India, 1800–1914". In *Health, Medicine, and Empire: Perspectives on Colonial India*, ed. Biswamoy Pati and Mark Harrison, 97–102. New Delhi: Orient Longman, 2001.

Greenough, Paul. "Variolation and Vaccination in South Asia, c.1700–1865: A Preliminary Note", *Social Science and Medicine* 14, 1980, 345–47.

Hacking, Ian. "Making Up People". In *The Science Studies Reader*, ed. Mario Biagioli, 161–71. New York and London: Routledge, 1999.

Hamilton, Sue. "From the Buddha to Buddhaghosa: Changing Attitude Toward the Human Body in Theravada Buddhism". In *Religious Reflections on the Human Body*, ed. Jane Marie Law, 46–61. Bloomington and Indianapolis: Indiana University Press, 1995.

Harrison, Mark. "Medicine and Orientalism: Perspectives on Europe's Encounter with Indian Medical Systems". In *Health, Medicine and Empire: Perspectives on Colonial India*, ed. Biswamoy Pati and Mark Harrison, 37–81. Hyderabad: Orient Longman, 2001.

——. "Disease, Diplomacy and International Commerce: The Origins of International Sanitary Regulation in the Nineteenth Century". *Journal of Global History* 1, 2006, 197–217.

Iijima, Wataru and Wakimura, Kohei. "Kindai Ajia ni okeru Teikoku syugi to Iryo Kosyu eisei". In *Sippei Kaihatsu Teikoku-iryo*, ed. Miichi Masatoshi, Saito Osamu, Wakimura Kohei, and Iijima Wataru, 75–95. Tokyo: Tokyo Daigaku Syuppan, 2001.

Ileto, Reynaldo C. "Cholera and the Origins of the American Sanitary Order in the Philippines". In *Imperial Medicine and Indigenous Societies*, ed. David Arnold, 125–48. Manchester and New York: Manchester University Press, 1988.

Kaur, Amarjit. "Indian Labour, Labour Standards, and Workers' Health in Burma and Malaya, 1900–1940". *Modern Asian Studies* 40, no. 2, 2006, 425–75.

Kelton, Paul. "Avoiding the Smallpox Spirits: Colonial Epidemics and Southeastern Indian Survival". *Ethnohistory* 51, no. 1, Winter 2004, 45–71.

Ko Ko, U Thaung, and Soe Aung. "Myanmar—General Perspectives". In *Conquest of Scourges in Myanmar*, 3–45. Yangon: Myanmar Academy of Medical Science, 2002.

Kumar, Deepak. "Unequal Contenders, Uneven Ground: Medical Encounters in British India, 1820–1920". In *Western Medicine as Contested Knowledge*, ed. Andrew Cunnigham and Bridie Andrews, 172–90. Manchester: Manchester University Press, 1997.

Latour, Bruno. "Give me a Laboratory and I Will Raise the World". In *The Science Studies Reader*, ed. Mark Biagioli, 258–75. New York and London: Routledge, 1999.

MacLeod, Roy. "Passage in Imperial Service: From Empire to Commonwealth". *Journal of World History* 4, no. 1, 1993, 117–50.

——. "On Visiting the 'Moving Metropolis' in Reflections on the Architecture of Imperial Science". *Historical Records of Australian Science* 5 (1982), 1–16.

MacNalty, A. S., and J. Craigie. "Sydney Arthur Monckton Copeman, 1862–1947", *Obituary Notices of Fellows of the Royal Society* 6, no. 17, November 1948, 37–50.

Maekawa, Kyutarou. "Bakin Nikki ni miru Edo no Toso syuzoku" [Prevailing Custom of Smallpox Treatment From the Diary of Bakin Takizawa.]. *Nihon Ishigaku Zasshi* 22, no. 4, October 1976, 47–61.

Matsuki, Akitomo. "'Roshia Gyuto Zensho' Ansei-ban no Syuppan no keii ni tuite" [On the Circumstances of the Publication of the 1855 Edition of 'Roshia Gyuto Zensho' (Russian Vaccination Book)]. *Nihon Ishigaku Zasshi* 45, no. 3, September 1999, 401–11.

Matsumoto, Naoki. "Kaei ni-nen no Syuto denrai to Sessu". In *Niho Yogaku-shi no Kenkyu III*, ed. Arisaka Takamichi, 237–50. Osaka: Sogen-sha, 1974.

Maung Shein. "State Investment in Burma Railways, 1874–1914". *Journal of the Burma Research Society* 44, no. 2, December 1961.

Min Naing, Maung. "Italians in the Service of Burmese Kings in Late Nineteenth Century". *Journal of the Burma Research Society* 62, nos. 1–2, December 1979, 177–213.

Mori, Osamu. "Inpaku ni okeru Gyuto Sessu no hajime" [The First Vaccination by Cowpox in Inaba and Hoki.]. In *Nihon Ishigaku Zasshi* 37, no. 4, October 1991), 513–33.

Najita, Tetsuo. "Ambiguous Encounters: Ogata Koan and International Studies in Late Tokugawa Osaka". In *Osaka: The Merchants' Capital of Early Modern Japan*, ed. James L. MaClain and Wakita Osamu, 213–42. Ithaca: Cornell University Press, 1999.

Naono, Atsuko. "Inoculators, the Indigenous Obstacle to Vaccination in Colonial Burma". In *Medicine in Colonial Myanmar*, ed. Monique Skidmore. Copenhagen: NIAS, forthcoming.

Naraindas, Harish. "Care, Welfare, and Treason: The Advent of Vaccination in the Nineteenth Century", *Contributions to Indian Sociology,* n.s., vol. 32, no. 1, 1998, 67–98.

Oki Akira. "*Yamai to Iyashi no Rekishi-Mou hitotsu no Indonesia-shi Kenkyu wo mezashite*" [The History of Disease and Healing in Indonesia: In Search of an Alternative Approach to Indonesian History]. *Tonan-Ajia Kenkyu* 34, no. 2, September 1996, 339–69.

Owen, Norman G. "Toward a History of Health in Southeast Asia". In *Death and Disease in Southeast Asia*, ed. Norman Owen, 3–30. Oxford: Oxford University Press, 1987.

Pickering, Andrew. "The Mangle of Practice: Agency and Emergnece in the Sociology of Science" In *The Science Studies Reader*, ed. Mario Biagioli, 372–93. New York and London: Routledge, 1999.

Polak, M. F. "Smallpox Control in Indonesia during the Second Quarter of the Century and Re-Establishment of Endemic Smallpox from 1947". *Tropical and Geographical Medicine* 20, September 1968, 243–50.

Porter, Dorothy. "Public Health". In *Companion Encyclopedia of the History of Medicine*, ed. W. F. Bynum and Roy Porter, 2: 1231–59. London: Routledge, 2001.

Porter, Dorothy, and Roy Porter. "The Politics of Prevention: Anti-Vaccinationism and Public Health in Nineteenth-Century England". *Medical History* 32, 1988, 231–52.

Ramasubban, Radhika. "Imperial Health in British India, 1857–1900". In *Disease, Medicine, and Empire: Perspectives on Western Medicine and the Experience of European Expansion*, ed. Roy Macleod and Milton Lewis, 38–60. London: Routledge, 1988.

Rosenberg, Charles E. "Introduction: Framing Disease: Illness, Society, and History". In *Framing Disease: Studies in Cultural History*, ed. Charles E. Rosenberg and Janet Golden, xiii–xxvi. New Brunswick: Rutgers University Press, 1997.

Rotermund, Hartmut O. "Demonic Affliction or Contagious Disease? Changing Perceptions of Smallpox in the Late Edo Period". *Japanese Journal of Religious Studies* 28, nos. 3–4, 2001, 373–98.

Sen Satadru. "Policing the Savage: Segregation, Labor, and State Medicine in the Andamans". *Journal of Asian Studies* 58, no. 3, August 1999, 753–73.

Silverstein, Josef. "Politics and Railroads in Burma and India", *JBRS* 45, no. 1, June 1962.

Sò-myín-hnín and Twet-aung. *Amyò-tha-yè-hnín-Myanmá-hsèi-binya-shin-myà*. Rangoon: Sapeibiman, 1998.

Thaung, U, and Ko Ko. "The Eradication of Smallpox". In *Conquest of Scourges in Myanmar*, ed. Ko Ko, Kyaw Lwin, and U Thaung, 47–119. Yangon: Myanmar Academy of Medical Science, 2002.

Worboys, Michael. "British Colonial Medicine and Tropical Imperialism: A Comparative Perspective". In *Dutch Medicine in the Malay Archipelago, 1816–1942*, ed. A. M. Luyendijk-Elshout, G. M. van Heteren, A. de Knecht-van Eekelen, and M. J. D. Poulissen, 153–68. Amsterdam: Rodopi, 1989.

——. "Manson, Ross and Colonial Medical Policy: Tropical Medicine". In *Disease, Medicine, and Empire: Perspectives on Western Medicine and the Experience of European Expansion*, ed. Roy Macleod and Milton Lewis, 21–37. London: Routledge, 1988.

Wujastyk, Dominik. "A Pious Fraud: The Indian Claims for Pre-Jennerian Smallpox Vaccination". In *Studies on Indian Medical History* 2, ed. G. J. Meulenbeld and Dominik Wujastyk, 131–67. Groningen: Egbert Forsten, 1987.

## Unpublished Conference Papers

Boomgaard, Peter. "Smallpox Vaccination in Troubled Times: 1913–1951", Paper prepared for the workshop 'Local Transmutations of Global Phenomena: An Historical Reassessment of Smallpox Prevention, Vaccination and the State', The Wellcome Trust Centre for the History of Medicine at UCL, London, 30 June–1 July 2006.

Tosa, Keiko. "Weiza Beliefs and Healing: Rituals for the Prevention of Disease and Disaster". Paper presented at the Burma Studies Conference in 2006.

## Unpublished Thesis

Naono, Atsuko. "The State of Vaccination: British Doctors, Indigenous Cooperation, and the Fight Against Smallpox in Colonial Burma". Ph.D. thesis. Ann Arbor: University of Michigan, 2005.

# Index

*New titles in the series*

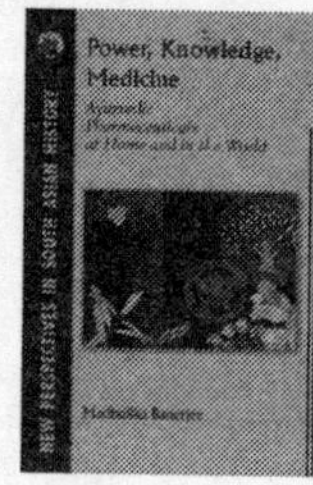


Power, Knowledge, Medicine: Ayurvedic Pharmaceuticals at Home and in the World
*Madhulika Banerjee*

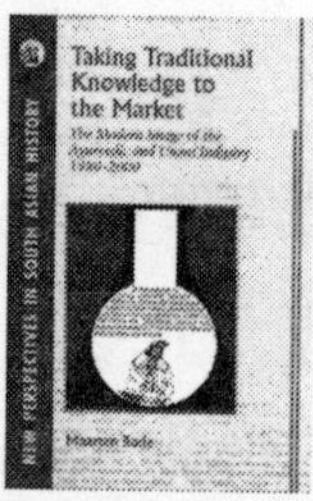


Taking Traditional Knowledge to the Market: The Modern Image of the Ayurvedic and Unani Industry, 1980–2000
*Maarten Bode*

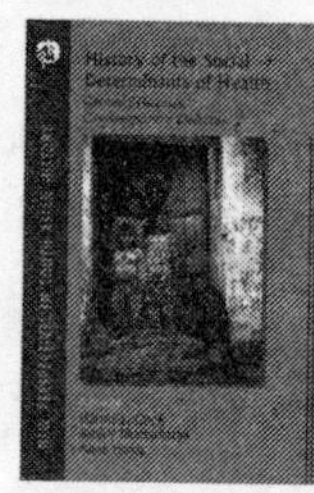

History of the Social Determinants of Health: Global Histories, Contemporary Debates
*Edited by*
*Harold J. Cook, Sanjoy Bhattacharya and Anne Hardy*

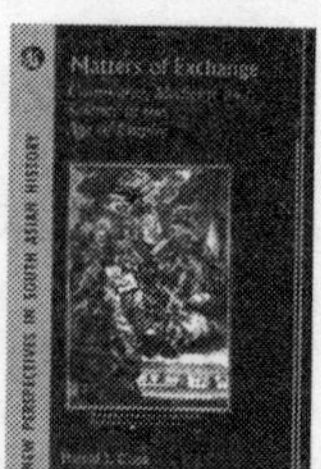


Matters of Exchange: Commerce, Medicine and Science in the Age of Empire
*Harold J. Cook*

*Forthcoming titles in the series*

Pathways of Empire: Circulation, 'Public Works' and Social Space in Colonial Orissa, c. 1780–1914
*Ravi Ahuja*

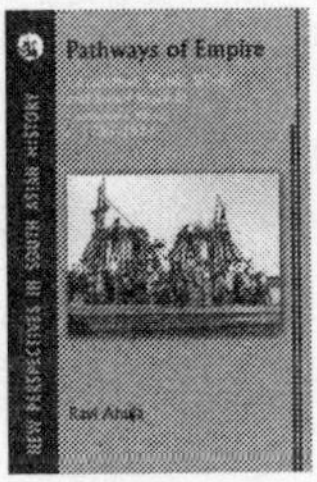


Against Stigma: Studies in Caste, Race and Justice since Durban
*Edited by*
*Balmurli Natrajan and Paul Greenough*

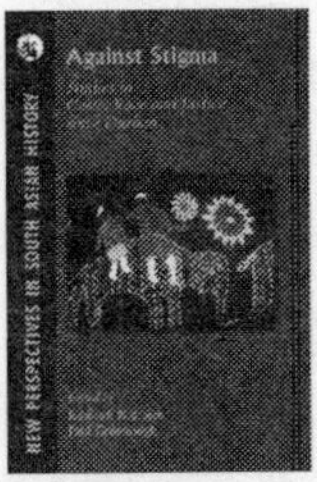


'Low and Licentious Europeans':
White Subalterns in Nineteenth-Century Colonial India
*Harald Fischer-Tiné*

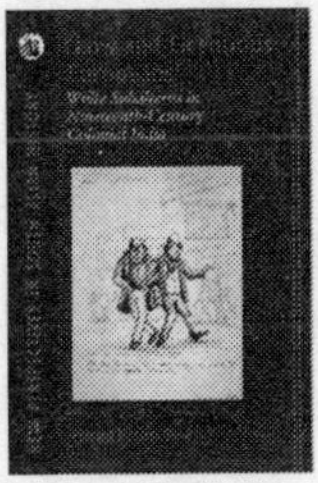